Eat to Beat Cancer

Eat to Beat Cancer

by J. Robert Hatherill, Ph.D.

RENAISSANCE BOOKS
Los Angeles

Library of Congress Cataloging-in-Publication Data

Hatherill, J. Robert.
    Eat to beat cancer / J. Robert Hatherill.
    p. cm.
    Includes bibliographical references and index.
    ISBN 1-58063-033-2 (alk. paper)
    1. Cancer—Nutritional aspects. 2. Cancer—Prevention.
    3. Cancer—Diet therapy. I. Title.
    RC268.45.H38 1998
    616.99'4052—dc21
    98-38397
    CIP

10 9 8 7 6 5 4 3 2 1

Design by Barbara Briggs Garibay

Distributed by St. Martin's Press
Manufactured in the United States of America
First Edition

This book is dedicated to my Uncle, Robert Theodore Morin,
who opened a young boy's eyes to the wonders of nature.

Contents

List of Figures

Acknowledgments

Many people were vital contributors to *Eat to Beat Cancer*. I am grateful to Eric Zimmerman for his support and suggestions throughout the creation of this book.

Dr. Rob Wilder and Dr. Mel Manalis provided critical comments of the manuscript.

I am indebted to Dr. Paul Volz, Dr. William Fennel, and Lee Lerner who years ago prepared me for the task of writing this book.

I am also indebted to Phil and Cindy Waldeck, Grant and Terry Adamson, Linda A. Rolfe, Anna M. Hatherill, Janet Patane, Eric and Denise Guempel, Juliane Kraus, Mike and Charlotte Beauchamp, Marty and Karen Lutz, Gordon and Marilyn Bigelow, and Angela Wells for their innumerable ideas and assistance.

My gratitude and thanks to the expert editorial talents of Richard F. X. O'Connor, Arthur Morey, and Jill Whitesides-Woo. Appreciation must also go to my agent Liz Ziemska, who was a vital part of this project and to my publisher Bill Hartley. Thanks also to Steve Brown for the illustrations and his help in designing the charts.

Why I Wrote This Book

Over the last twenty years a mystifying number of my friends and relatives, including even young children, have developed nervous system disorders, cancer, or heart disease. The most tragic story for me was learning that the father of my best friend suffered from cancer. I had never met a kinder, gentler person in my life. Throughout the illness my friend sent me detailed accounts of his father's relentless, painful disease. Though this gentleman received the finest medical attention, he missed the joys of having grandchildren and died at the age of fifty-nine. I was shocked to learn of his death and was shocked again a few years later when my friend's wife lost her own father to cancer.

In recent years cancer diagnosis and treatment procedures have improved, but the vast majority of cancers still lack effective treatments. The choices still involve some form of surgery, radiation, or chemotherapy. Unfortunately, these often cause side effects more severe than the disease.

For all these reasons, I became interested in researching the underlying causes of cancer and heart disease. As I began this inquiry it surprised me to learn that many foods are full of natural chemicals that can trigger cancer. Cancer is also linked to compounds that are produced normally in the body, such as bile acids. How can you avoid infusions of bile acids produced by your own liver? It also seemed impossible to prevent exposure to dietary carcinogens unless you stopped eating altogether.

A fresh, completely different approach to the disease was needed, and I took exceptional interest in anything that might promise illness prevention. The foundations of a new field of prevention—*chemoprevention*—had already been formed; the concept that natural substances found in whole fresh foods could provide powerful weapons against cancer, and against other chronic ailments as well. Today exciting new scientific evidence to support chemoprevention is growing.

The thrilling implications of these recent discoveries have convinced me that practicing a "chemopreventive" lifestyle can save millions of lives. This is not another far-reaching health claim. Countless scientific studies have shown positive results.

Chemo*prevention* is not chemo*therapy*. It is a therapeutic breakthrough, and it will become the most exciting field of science in the 21st century. I firmly believe that becoming knowledgeable about chemoprevention will offer protection from the ravages of cancer and numerous other illnesses. This book will make you aware of those many benefits.

Cancer, a Mutiny of Your Cells

Cancer is the most dreaded foe of modern medicine. Yet it is not our most lethal enemy, since death occurs more frequently through heart disease. Cancer has the reputation of a merciless torturer inflicting slow, painful death. A cancerous cell is a battle-hardened warrior, and when a cancer cell starts a mutiny it happens like this.

A solitary cell from among your over fifty trillion cells transforms into a cancerous one. This does not happen overnight. Through the decades the cell has been pelted with too many mutations, repeatedly exposed to toxic chemicals, and it has been ordered to divide on cue until exhaustion has set in. Every cell has a breaking point, and at that point the cancer cell starts its war. But how can this solitary cancer cell cause so much havoc to the other fifty trillion normal cells? The mutinous cell defies all the orders that the normal cells obey. Over ten years or so it divides and divides, giving birth to a small army of new cancer cells. Yet this mutinous tumor mass may be barely perceptible to you.

Initial detection of many types of tumor depends upon its location. If encamped in the skin, cancerous cells will be quickly discovered, and surgery is usually successful.

If a cancer is entrenched in the lung, cells churn out new members slowly, expanding their numbers. In order to sustain growth, the tumor builds an independent blood supply. To invade otherwise healthy territories it has to penetrate cell barriers, which it does by elaborating special protein-degrading substances. It can take decades for a mass of tumor cells to overcome these obstacles.

On the other hand, daily infusions of chemopreventives through whole foods will cause the tumor cells to remain in an arrested stage of growth. Most people in industrialized countries consume diets that are weak in cancer slashing agents, a practice that gives the tumor time to grow. During this period of the tumor's daunting expansion you may feel fine. At most you have a pesky cough or maybe an unexplained bout with pneumonia. Meanwhile the cancer cells are embroiled in a *blitzkrieg*-style invasion.

A routine chest X-ray may then show an "area of concern." Further analysis confirms suspicions that you are harboring a malignant growth in your lung. Determined to fight the cancer, you employ the best team of cancer physicians, who discuss your strategy and options. They decide the best course of action is to surgically strike the large tumor. Then if the entire population of cancer cells can be surgically removed, you deliver a *coup de grace*.

Of course you are relieved that the primary cell mass has been removed—until later diagnostic reports indicate massive widespread invasions of distant tissue sites. Once again the cancer team meets and discusses countermeasures. You try chemotherapy and radiation treatments, but they're astonishingly ineffective against your cancer, and they're also destructive to your healthy cells and tissues. Heated debate ensues among your cancer team. Finally a trusted physician mirrors your concerns, confiding that the cancer cells have infiltrated and established themselves strategically in most organ systems. One doctor proclaims that further countermeasures will only increase your pain and suffering. In essence, your team stares at another humiliating defeat.

What follows in this book is the latest scientific information on a natural defense, a missing link in our understanding of disease prevention. Cancer *prevention* has turned out to be a powerful and effective approach. You can *Eat to Beat Cancer*!

Introduction

One hundred years ago our bucolic ancestors grew and took most of their sustenance from fresh fruits, grains, and vegetables. Meat and other animal products were costly and in short supply. Farming was a cottage industry in which fertile fields were carefully replenished with composted plants and animal manure, and crops were harmoniously rotated. In these humbler times people rarely got cancer. In fact, heart disease was so rare that medical textbooks from the mid- to late 1800s failed to include it.

The doctor of the future will give no medicine, but will interest his patients in the care of the human frame, in diet, and in the cause and prevention of disease.

—Thomas Edison 1847–1931

Something has gone fundamentally wrong in present times, as heart disease and cancer have emerged as the two most vexing killers in affluent countries. Dramatic changes did not occur overnight in the Western diet but have been instituted gradually over the last one hundred years.

Progress first burst forth with the supplanting of plow horses by tractors. A team of horses could prepare several acres for planting in one day; tractors plowed fifty acres a day. Horses, which were no longer used for plowing, became a measurement of an engine's power. This progress was heralded as a great boon to the growth of farming. The fertile heartland soil was turned into a mechanized industrial complex, employing oil-based fertilizers and pesticides to boost crop yields. In fact, America developed into the largest farming economy in the world. And World War II prosperity replaced time-honored diets. Fat-laden animal products lacking fiber and other critical anticancer agents took the place of fresh, fiber-rich, plant-based foods. Animal edibles started to dominate the nation's dinner plates.

The refinement of food came along in the late 1800s with the use of roller mills to process grains. By that century's end, the canning industry was blanching food with heat prior to sealing it up in metal tins. During the 1950s and 1960s, widespread refinements to foods became common as prosperity delivered new and complex food-processing factories. As television became embedded in the American lifestyle, food companies responded with fattening snack foods and frozen TV dinners. Highly processed, overcooked meals could be swiftly made to order while watching your favorite sitcom. Life seemed good.

But processed foods stripped away all unnecessary fiber, and they did not provide adequate nutrition. Breads were so depleted of fiber that a whole loaf could be crushed by hand into the size of a baseball. To limit bacteria that would cause spoilage, foods were heated to excessive temperatures in processing. But the high heat also destroyed natural anticancer agents, forming potent cancer-producing chemicals in the process. To tantalize our palates and to halt food from spoiling, food makers began tinkering with thousands of additives.

Finally, eager American food companies changed the very nature of food's purpose. Rather than valuing it for its ability to sustain health, food became an object of chic fashion statements, representing identity with trendy market icons and celebrities rather than nurturing health.

Then friends started dying too young, from heart disease and cancer. At the time few people thought about diet's relationship to disease. Over time cancer and heart disease have become, tragically, normal parts of life.

During the 1970s a British researcher, Denis Burkitt, traveled to rural Africa where he reported a cluster of people who had escaped colon and large intestine cancer because of their high-fiber diet. Did this imply that eating fiber-poor convenience foods increased cancer rates? At the time no one placed any blame. Yet this discovery caused the American people to become more occupied with their intake of dietary fiber.

Concurrently, individuals started to realize that high levels of cholesterol were associated with heart disease. It became clear that saturated fats were linked to heart disease and to cancer. Then polyunsaturated fats and environmental pollutants began to be accused of promoting cancer.

The carefree days of the American TV dinner were long gone. Perhaps they were convenient, but they had enormous health consequences. Nevertheless, catchy commercials and enticing, well-financed marketing schemes still tempted us with foods that were bad for us.

In the 1980s we learned about the dangers of eating fat-laden foods. Simultaneously, death from heart disease—still the most lethal disorder—started to level off, perhaps due to widespread installation of emergency coronary care units and to the discovery of new, improved medications.

Meanwhile cancer rates during these decades skyrocketed to the highest point in world history, catching the attention of American leaders who felt compelled to become involved. After signing the 1971 National Cancer Act, Richard Nixon defiantly bragged that America would cure cancer within five years. This galvanized the search for cancer cures through a massive taxpayer-funded research program. The most brilliant scientific minds were charged with unraveling the mysteries of cancer and, since 1971, over $35 billion has been invested in cancer research.

As the country was celebrating the Bicentennial in 1976, five years after the National Cancer Act was signed, a pattern emerged in the research. More people had cancer or were hobbled by chronic illnesses than the year before.

How was this possible? America had pioneered the complex technology to land a human on the moon, and we seemed to have the most sophisticated medical science system on the face of the globe. Yet with all cancer statistics tallied, despite the multibillion-dollar war against cancer, people were developing cancer at a higher rate than ever before.

Today people are living longer with cancer. But does a decreased death rate measure quality of life for individuals suffering from cancer?

Why did America lose its hard-fought battle against cancer? Is cancer a more tenacious opponent than we originally assumed? Do we need to spend more money?

The answer is unwittingly heard in sweaty locker rooms around the country, drilled into players by every football coach: The best offense is a strong defense.

There is no denying that many major illnesses have not been contained by offensive treatments. To this day, polio and smallpox cannot be treated successfully once you have them. Only a preventive, defensive approach has proved effective, as the use of vaccinations dramatically suppressed these diseases. Many illnesses, including cancer, cannot be treated or cured as easily as they can be prevented, by changes in diet.

Overall, stomach, rectal, uterine, and cervical cancers are on the decline. However, the incidence rate for all other cancers has risen steadily since 1950.

In young men testicular cancer is increasing. Prostate cancer increased 266 percent between 1950 and 1992, becoming the number one cancer for men. Lung and skin cancer are thriving. Malignant melanoma, an aggressive and deadly form of skin cancer, zoomed up almost 400 percent among whites between 1950 and 1992. Today, for unknown reasons, breast cancer is the most common cancer found in women who live in industrialized countries, and its incidence is escalating. If current trends for breast cancer continue, by the year 2000 cancer will be the biggest killer in the United States. The cancer rate is showing no signs of going down, and there has been an onslaught of new nervous and immune system disorders.

No one knows why cancer and other illnesses are becoming so prevalent, though crucial environmental factors are clearly at play. Pioneering research suggests accelerating statistics are probably the result of toxic changes in our environment, and are due to more effective methods of diagnosis as well. Mounting evidence certainly suggests that a variety of ailments are linked to environmental chemicals and to dietary factors. Undeniably, our polluted environment plays a critical role in causing cancer.

Amazingly, illness prevention has received very little attention as a treatment method. In America's battle against cancer, defense is painfully absent. Medical science has developed a fully stocked offensive arsenal of surgery, radiation, and chemotherapy. But it tends to ignore the potential of prevention as the best cure.

Traditionally the focus of medicine has been on intervention and the management of diseases—highly skilled techniques to manage and treat symptoms, such as pain or high blood pressure. To combat cancer and chronic illness, billions of dollars have been dedicated to equipment that can diagnose the presence of disease. Yet modern medicine has put relatively little emphasis on prevention.

This is not surprising. There is meager profit in disease prevention. Medicine is a fee-for-service industry, and it's much faster and certainly more profitable to administer a sophisticated diagnostic test than it is to educate someone on a preventive diet and lifestyle. A fifteen-minute MRI scan can cost $800 to $2,000. A physician could hardly justify charging this much to chat for fifteen minutes about illness prevention.

For decades the American medical establishment has largely ignored preventive medicine. Perhaps this explains why people are clamoring for alternatives to modern medicine. It is a tragic paradox that diet, probably the single most crucial factor in disease, plays only a minor role in medical education.

Unfortunately, detection has been masquerading as prevention. Generations of physicians have extolled the benefits of cancer detection, promoting breast, skin, and testicular self-examination as if they were methods of prevention. Detection comes in many forms: mammograms or X-rays for breast cancer, prostate-specific antigen (PSA) tests, digital rectal exams for prostate cancer, Pap smears for cervical cancer, and ultrasonography, which is an imaging instrument used to detect some cancers. Standard tools of the trade include endoscopy, used to examine the esophagus and stomach; and sigmoidoscopy and colonoscopy, procedures for observing the colon.

Everyone agrees that sensitive techniques to detect cancer do save lives. The sooner you detect a tumor, the more able you are to remove it. The three primary cancer treatments—surgery, radiation, and chemotherapy—are more successful and effective if a primary tumor has not invaded other locations. And once you detect a mass of cancer cells, no matter how small, it is certainly far too late to start prevention.

The fact is, however, that the most sophisticated and sensitive cancer detection equipment cannot detect a tumor until it has churned out over 1 billion cells and weighs around 1 gram. More likely the cancer cells will need to multiply to about 10 billion strong before they are able to be unmasked by most imaging equipment. By this time most tumors weigh close to 10 grams. Only ten more cell doublings and the tumor will reach the size of a small watermelon and weigh 2.2 pounds! The vast majority (about 75 percent) of the cancer's life

CHANGES IN RATE OF CANCER				
CANCER TYPE	INCIDENCE IN 1992	DEATHS IN 1992	INCIDENCE % CHANGE SINCE 1950[1]	DEATHS % CHANGE SINCE 1950[1]
stomach	24,400	13,630	−74.8	−77.6
cervix	13,500	4,641	−76.6	−74.5
rectum	45,000	7,785	−21.3	−66.9
colon	111,000	49,204	+21.6	−15.0
larynx	12,500	3,966	+50.9	−7.4
testicles	6,300	355	+113.6	−69.6
bladder	51,600	10,705	+57.1	−34.8
Hodgkin's disease	7,400	1,639	+17.3	−67.8
childhood cancer	7,800	1,679	+4.9	−62.4
leukemia	28,200	19,417	+8.7	−2.1
thyroid	12,500	1,111	+115.3	−49.5
ovaries	21,000	13,181	+5.2	+2.5
lung	168,000	145,801	+267.4	+264.0
skin melanoma	32,000	6,568	+393.3	+155.0
breast	180,000	43,063	+55.9	+0.2
prostate	132,000	34,238	+266.4	+20.7
kidney	26,500	10,427	+120.6	+37.2
liver	15,400	9,554	+107.3	+22.8
non-Hodgkin's lymphoma	41,000	20,058	+183.6	+123.1
multiple myeloma	12,500	9,247	+235.8	+194.0
brain	16,900	11,941	+85.2	+50.4
pancreas	28,300	26,070	+13.6	+17.8
all types excluding lung	962,000	374,747	+40.8	−15.0
all types	1,130,000	520,548	+54.3	+9.6

[1] 1950 to 1992. From SEER *Cancer Statistics Review* 1973–1992. NIH publication 96-2789. National Cancer Institute, 1995. Table I-3, pg. 17 (U.S. Cancer Incidence and Deaths in 1992, and the Percent Change in Age-Adjusted Rates of Incidence and Death per 100,000 U.S. Population 1950–1992).

occurs before the cancer is clinically detectable by even the most sophisticated detection techniques.

Oddly, until now cancer has been treated as an end stage, or as a single event that leads to the destruction or the removal of tumors. However, although cancer may appear to strike suddenly, often without warning, it does not just happen overnight. Rather, it is a slow, steady progression that takes twenty, thirty, even forty years to reveal itself. A cancer diagnosis is one step in a decades-long process that has resulted in a tumor that may be barely detectable to the touch (and this is most apt to occur if the tumor is on frequently touched skin). Current methods of cancer detection do make it possible to search for and destroy these tumors sooner, but they offer nothing to prevent them in the first place.

Cancer develops over a lifetime. Effective countermeasures should be employed over your entire life, with lines of defense formed ten to twenty years before a cancer might become detectable. This is a vital lesson in reducing cancer rates. Long before you discover a rebel army of mutinous cells, you can be preventing a battle with cancer!

Stopping Cancer in Time

Understanding the timeline for cancer is crucial in suggesting methods for its prevention. Most cancers have a ten- or twenty-year interval between their carcinogenic stimulus and the appearance of a thriving tumor. The importance of diet cannot be stressed enough.

Chemopreventive agents in whole fresh foods can slow, interrupt, or even reverse the course of cancer. Many of these agents have been shown to stop normal cells from becoming rebel cancer cells, and some will actually even reverse cancer cells back into normal cells.

The best defense against cancer is two-pronged: actively ingesting chemopreventive agents in food, and avoiding cancer-inducing substances in the first place. As the details of chemoprevention become widely known, this will become heralded as the most viable way to win the war against cancer. A gram of chemoprevention is worth a kilogram of cure.

People often envision cancer as a single disease, like diabetes. However, cancer is actually over 150 diseases (perhaps upwards of 300) and can arise in any organ or tissue in the body. The vast majority of cancers arise in tissues that are in contact with the environment, or they arise where cells are actively dividing (such as in the lungs, large intestine, and breasts).

Cells are normally dividing all over your body. Why is there a greater likelihood of cancer arising in tissues that are dividing? Part of cellular protection lies in the fact that when the cell is not dividing, its DNA (deoxyribonucleic acid) is tightly bunched together like a super-compressed spring. When a cell divides the DNA uncoils, exposing a larger surface area for potential damage. Also, the act of cell division is prone to errors which can lead to permanent alterations of DNA.

Mutation

A deeper cause of cancer is an obscure event called mutation, a process where DNA is despoiled by mistakes. When the mistakes are savage enough the cell cannot control growth, so it multiplies and invades other parts of the body. Even if the cause of the mutation is suddenly removed—for instance, even if you stop smoking—the cancer cells continue to huddle together and keep growing.

When a cell is in the act of dividing it is more sensitive to mutation or to alteration of genetic information, because while the cell is preparing to divide, less energy is directed to the systems that repair DNA. The DNA repair systems scan and repair small errors in the entire length of DNA and function as natural defenses against a number of cancers. Prolonged cell division can cause mutations or defects in the genetic material called DNA.

For example, the sweetener saccharin has been linked to cancer. It caused bladder cancer in rats by stimulating cell division. When you have a condition of prolonged cell division, you are more likely to find cancer.

It is also known that certain intestinal bacteria can activate substances such as bile and ingested fats to become cancer-producing chemicals, or carcinogens. Over time, for example, carcinogens

TISSUE SITES WHERE MOST CANCERS ARISE

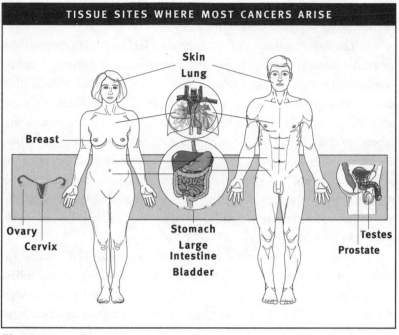

Figure 1

increase cell division and change the surface of the colon. These changes may eventually lead to cancer. The DNA of a normal cell has been permanently altered into a cancer cell.

The majority of cells found in the adult brain and in nervous tissue do not divide. For that reason, any damage to the nervous system becomes irreversible. A cancer that originates in the brain or nervous tissue is rare, and in fact is usually only seen in infants. Adult brain tumors have usually originated in another location, then spread through the blood, lodging in the brain. Brain cancer comprises only 2 percent of total cancers.

Studies have confirmed that 92 percent of all cancers arise from surface cells (epithelia) that are directly in contact with environmental factors. It is within these tissues where cells are actively dividing that most cancer is born. Certain cancer sites, such as the large intestine, are more frequently affected than others. Almost half of all deaths from cancer result from lung, large intestine, and breast cancers.

The causes of cancer follow a diverse series of events appearing in commonly accepted developmental stages.

The first insult usually comes from a DNA-altering chemical or virus. An insult to the DNA may also be inherited from your parents, predisposing you to cancer. In either case, cells that receive this molecular peppering are said to be *initiated*. These initiated cells are believed to remain silent until they are *promoted*. Promoters are substances that signal the DNA of the initiated cells to be read. When the altered message is read, this may lead to uncontrolled cell division or to a cancerous cell. Initiation can be thought of as starting the engine; promotion as placing the transmission in drive. This is the widely accepted two-step model of cancer. If either initiation or promotion are inhibited, cancer will be prevented.

In exploring cancer we find that all expressions of the disease share one common factor: The cells have acquired uncontrolled growth. In order to better understand cells, let's consider the analogy of a train. The DNA of a cell acts like a train track, guiding cells along their course. As the train track deteriorates from the influence of cancer-producing chemicals, chances of derailment become likely. A runaway train or one that jumps the tracks becomes cancer—a mass of cells that have lost control and are spreading throughout an otherwise healthy body.

When normal cells contact one another, one of the first things that happens is that they turn off cell division. This is called *contact inhibition*. Cancerous cells, on the other hand, have lost this critical feature of contact inhibition, so when they contact adjacent cells they continue to multiply. When cancer cells reach ample numbers they break free and start to invade surrounding tissues. They even colonize distant sites by entering blood vessels, spreading cancer growths to other areas of the body.

Many believe that genetics play the most significant role in the development of cancer. But statistics show that genetics accounts for only 5 percent of all cancers. Overwhelming evidence suggests that environmental factors, not genetics or heredity, play the biggest role in the development of cancer and chronic disease.

Different countries have different "fingerprints" of cancer types. For instance, Japan has the highest rate of stomach cancer, while in the

U.S. colon and prostate cancer are very common. If cancer was mainly related to genetics, common sense says that Japanese who immigrate to the U.S. would retain high rates of stomach cancer. However, this does not occur. Japanese immigrants living in the United States have less stomach cancer but increased colon cancer, as is typical of Americans. Successive Japanese-American generations manifest even less stomach cancer and instead develop greater rates of colon and prostate cancer, thus reflecting cancer patterns for the American population.

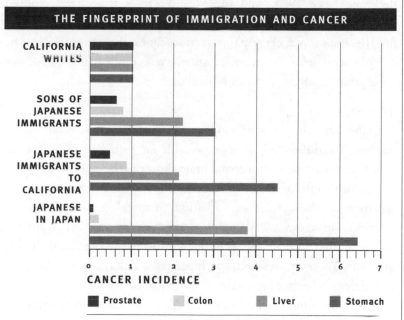

THE FINGERPRINT OF IMMIGRATION AND CANCER

CANCER INCIDENCE

Prostate   Colon   Liver   Stomach

Figure 2   Cancer has a characteristic fingerprint that follows people wherever they move in the world. Over time the fingerprint changes to fit the new country.

Cancer and Longevity

Some scientists dismiss cancer as a disease of aging since it appears more frequently in older people. After all, as time goes by, the more often your DNA will have sustained errors.

In prehistoric times humans tended to live about twenty-six years. But through the centuries average life expectancy has increased. At the turn of the century, life expectancy was about fifty years. Now in the United States it is between seventy and seventy-five years. Japan has the longest life expectancy on the planet, about eighty years.

Now let's suppose that the twenty-five-year increase in life expectancy in the U.S. during this century can be attributed to advances in medical technology, public health, immunizations, and reduced infant mortality. Then why do so many Americans fail to reach their life expectancy of seventy years? Heart disease and cancer are the two diseases that keep us from living to our potential. About 70 percent of deaths in the United States are caused by heart disease, cancer, and stroke. The good news is that heart disease has been declining since 1960. And some cancer rates have been reduced through early diagnosis, improved cancer therapies, and changes in lifestyle. Even so, cancer remains a serious illness that strikes nearly one out of every three Americans. Cancer, even if eventually cured, is a debilitating, costly, and painful disease.

Treatment

Two independent lines of evidence suggest that cancer detection methods themselves might be responsible for a number of increasing cancers, such as breast cancer and brain cancer in the elderly. Radiation is a known cause of breast cancer. Since breast tissues are exquisitely sensitive to the effects of radiation, medical X-rays, including mammograms, can translate into increased cancer. CAT scans are routinely used to diagnose abnormalities in many organs, including the brain. Yet recent research has suggested a link between CAT scans and increased brain cancer rates.

Many of our treatments for cancer are outdated and ineffective. For example, radiation treatments have been used to retard tumor growth, yet radiation therapy can trigger cancer in previously undisturbed areas. If you survive the initial cancerous attack, brace yourself. A New England Journal of Medicine study found that women who were given radiation treatment and survived early Hodgkin's cancers were 75 times more apt to develop breast cancer by age 45.[1]

The variety of agents used for treating cancer are actually toxic, lethal chemicals. Ideally, chemotherapy and radiation would commit molecular carnage only to cancer cells. Instead, severe toxicity is

---

[1] S. Bhatia, et al., Breast Cancer and Other Second Neoplasms after Childhood Hodgkin's Disease. N Engl J Med, 1996; 334:745–51.

incited in otherwise healthy tissue. Chemotherapy douses many healthy cells with molecular damage; it creates mutations, and by doing so, it increases the risk of future cancers. Infusions of cancer-fighting drugs are certainly more taxing to your health than taking a round of antibiotics.

As if this were not enough, painful surgical procedures that are used to remove cancerous growths can also spread cancer. Because most tumors are interlaced with blood vessels, cutting into the area frees tumor cells to move into otherwise healthy tissue, thereby risking the eruption of future cancers.

Since our current treatments are so dangerous, what should an individual with cancer do? You can't vaccinate children against cancer. And pills or lotions won't cure it.

Well let's consider again where cancer comes from. Of course a predisposition to cancer can be inherited from parents. But a number of landmark studies have independently estimated that up to ninety percent of cancer originates from the environment.

There are countless reasons why a cell may turn cancerous. Smoking is a factor that may cause about 30 percent of cancer deaths. Diet is the most important factor (60 percent). Other environmental risks include a bewildering array of chemicals and other occupational hazards, viruses, sun exposure, and radiation.

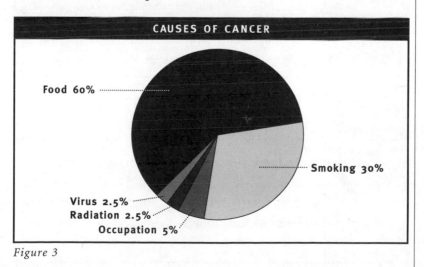

CAUSES OF CANCER

Food 60%

Smoking 30%

Virus 2.5%
Radiation 2.5%
Occupation 5%

Figure 3

Luckily, there is overwhelming scientific evidence that most cancers can be prevented.

In the last twenty years, a staggering amount of scientific information has clearly shown that certain compounds in food can provide significant protection against heart disease, toxicity, and cancer. A number of chronic illnesses, including heart disease, share some of the same underlying causes as cancer. For many years it was thought that cancer and heart disease were misfortunes that you

SUPER EIGHT FOOD GROUPS	
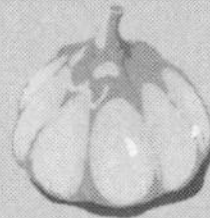	**1. Onion Group**—onion, garlic, asparagus
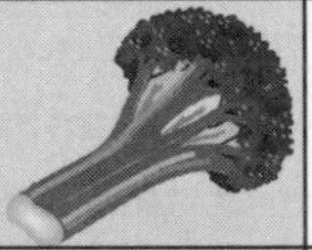	**2. Cruciferous Group**—broccoli, cabbage, cauliflower
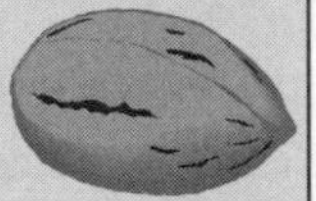	**3. Nuts & Seeds**—pumpkin seeds, sesame seeds, walnuts
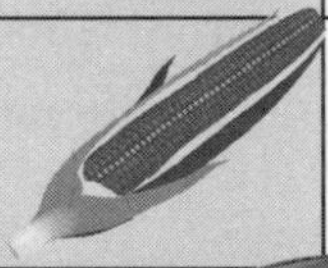	**4. Grass Group**—corn, oats, rice, wheat
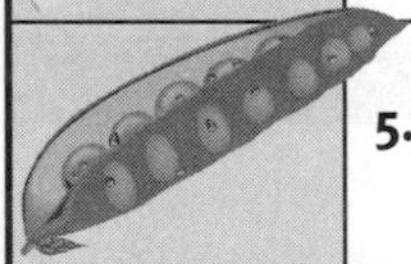	**5. Legume Group**—soybeans (tofu), green and wax beans, peas
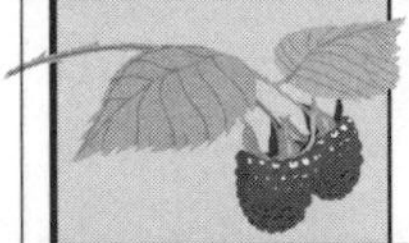	**6. Fruit**—citrus fruits, berries
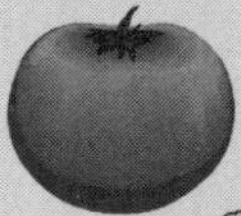	**7. Solanace Group**—tomatoes, potatoes
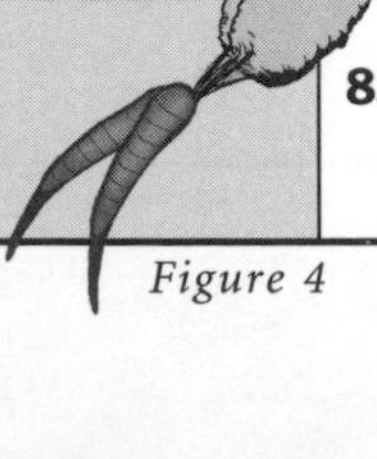	**8. Umbelliferous Group**—carrots, celery

Figure 4

braced for in later life and simply learned to accept. However, research shows that we don't have to sit back and wait as helpless victims.

Fresh fruits and vegetables provide a veritable feast of thousands of substances that you simply cannot get from eating processed food or by taking pills. Natural plant agents, or phytochemicals, have been meticulously crafted by plants for millions of years in response to stresses like drought, extreme temperatures, plant-eating insects, and intense sunlight. This exclusive group of plant compounds holds the secret of good health and forms the basis of the Super Eight Food Groups, which will be discussed in chapter 5. The Super Eight Food Groups were protecting animals long before bands of our apelike ancestors appeared on, and began roaming, the Serengeti plains. Modern-day cancer is actually a maladjusted response to present-day diets which lack these diverse, health-sustaining agents.

Consuming foods in all eight of the Super Eight Food Groups is like putting on a sturdy suit of anticancer body armor. Each food group that is absent from your diet eliminates a crucial shield. Each part of the armor provides an exclusive form of defense that is not duplicated by other segments, and the whole is greater than the sum of its parts. The Super Eight Food Groups are unique and are not duplicated by other food groups.

• • •

Rigorous scientifically controlled studies from around the globe support the principles brought forth in this book. These theories have been tried and tested, and they are supported by tens of thousands of research articles that affirm: *What you eat is a major determinate in heart disease and cancer—the most common causes of premature death* (see appendix A).

It's important to note that the insights contained in this book are not a "quick fix" or cure-all for existing health problems. Although the benefits of applying these principles are immediate, the information in this book does not replace the need for proper healthcare. Even very healthy people need medical services occasionally. *Eat to Beat Cancer* should be seen as an aid to lessen dependence on healthcare systems in the long term, simply by promoting a more healthful life style.

Current day diets have become dysfunctional largely because of processed and synthetic foods. This book can help you convert your diet into a defensive, anticancer solution. Throughout these pages you will be given practical techniques for solving the health problems that arise from eating a Western diet. Some examples will validate what you already know through common sense. *Eat to Beat Cancer* has identified the most protective, beneficial foods from around the globe and placed them in one simple, straightforward diet.

One great advantage of this cancer-busting regimen is that your food can taste just as good as ever. You don't have to learn to eat weird herbs or strange mushrooms; in fact, chocolate, red wine, and licorice can be part of the regimen! Also, with *Eat to Beat Cancer* you don't have to restructure your diet entirely. If you must have those ball-park hot dogs, just make sure you take an extra dose of vitamin C in order to block the formation of the cancer-causing chemicals used in cured meats.

No matter what your age, eating from the Super Eight Food Groups will improve your quality of life, health, and longevity.

Our Chemical Environment

The industrial revolution ushered in massive dependence on artificial chemicals for the first time in the history of our planet. These synthetically manufactured chemicals are now heavily relied upon, being used in an onslaught of consumer products such as pesticides, fertilizers, pigments, plastics, solvents, and synthetic fiber products. By the mid 1980s the National Research Council estimated that a whopping 5 million chemical compounds had been made by various chemical industries. In 1940, the manufacture of synthetic chemicals and chemicals for energy production in the U.S. was only 1/2 billion kilograms. That mushroomed to 173 billion kilograms by 1989.

Men dig their graves with their own teeth and die more by those fated instruments than the weapons of their enemies.
—Thomas Moffett, 1553–1604

Toxics

Every year more than 1,000 new and exotic chemicals are added to a current stockpile of 60,000 to 70,000 industrially marketed chemicals. Apparently we have so many chemicals that no one knows for sure how many are actually in use. Industry and automobiles have burned oceans of fossil fuel into by-products such as heavy metals that have been spewing from smokestacks and exhaust pipes, recasting the very surface of our planet. As a consequence of human activities the composition of the earth's crust has been permanently altered for the worse. And certainly the widespread use of these industrial chemicals has revised our bodies' internal chemistry as well.

You may find this statistic unbelievable. But it is now possible to detect over 600 different chemicals in our bodies that were not present in any human being before the early 1900s! If you think these chemicals are not betraying our health, think again.

The Bad News
- Cancer, stroke, and birth defects are increasing.
- Immune system and reproductive disorders are escalating.

- Nervous system disorders are flourishing.
- Learning disorders are skyrocketing.
- Infectious diseases are rising.

A Return to the Dark Ages?

If you were about to enter a darkened room, would you run at full speed to find a light switch? Of course not, but this is precisely what we are doing with many of the chemicals we're using in commerce. Today, for the sake of a burgeoning chemical industry, our health is being compromised. We have not fully characterized the toxicity of these chemicals, yet we are exposed to many of them in our food, air, and water. It is not your choice whether to participate; everyone on the planet is exposed and part of a massive experiment. Unfortunately this experiment is not controlled, making meaningful results or conclusions fraught with extreme difficulty.

If you look at the origin of many of our chronic nervous system illnesses, it's not surprising to find that they correlate with widespread chemical pollution. We have begun to notice that this alien chemical alteration is hostile to many life forms. Many wildlife creatures have disappeared since they cannot tolerate some of the human-induced changes. In Yosemite National Park seven species of amphibians are disappearing, and three have disappeared entirely. The chemical dusting of our planet has created new, often perplexing health hazards and illnesses. The environmental consequences are more apparent and more alarming every year.

Suppose, somehow, that a wise international agency were capable of putting an end to environmental contamination, as of now. Imagine eliminating global pollution in one fell swoop. Let's suppose that tomorrow we hear miraculous news that nations have banded together and adopted a zero discharge policy on the release of toxic chemicals. This would certainly be good news, and many might actually believe that our planet can quickly return to a pristine state. Hardly! Even if we totally cease releasing pollutants into the environment today, they are so persistent that they will accompany us well into the future. Therefore to fend off a polluted world, it is humans who must adapt to and accommodate this alien change in our environment.

For example, a deadly triad of metals—cadmium, lead, and mercury—persists almost indefinitely. Nature does not know how to deal with them. Cadmium and lead have been released into the environment largely through human activities.

GREENLAND ICE CAP[1]	
YEAR	LEAD LEVELS
880 B.C.	0.0005 mg/kg[2]
1750	0.01 mg/kg
1980s	0.21 mg/kg

[1] Autos and industry have caused a more than 400 times increase of lead in Greenland ice, since 880 B.C.

[2] mg/kg = milligrams of lead per kilogram of ice.

Pollution of the Body

Are these pollutants causing problems in humans? Every cancer researcher agrees that a considerable number of environmental pollutants cause budding mammary tumors in lab animals. Women exposed to PCBs or to DDT show increased breast cancer rates. In Florida, alligators have penises so short they cannot fertilize female alligators. In California, lesbian gulls on Santa Barbara Island resulted when low levels of DDT were introduced into gull eggs.

Environmental chemicals show the same kinds of results in altering male reproductive processes. PCBs are linked to a 50 percent reduction in sperm counts during the last half-century in men from industrialized countries! A study in Taiwan showed that males exposed to PCBs while in their mothers' wombs developed smaller penises when they matured, compared to normal Taiwanese males. These studies seem to confirm that PCB exposure in the womb may have more drastic results than exposure later in life.

Pesticides and other chemical residues are easy targets since many chemicals that have been banned have received high-profile press coverage. It is easy to concede increases in cancer to the use of pesticides and chemicals.

However, a number of chemicals are also potent immune system poisons. A study conducted with harbor seals has shown that seals fed fish with higher pollutant levels consistently showed more infections and immune system dysfunction. Our behavior is so easily influenced by toxic chemicals that in the 1980s, a brand new discipline called *behavioral toxicology* came into existence.

Birth defects are also increasing. The Centers for Disease Control reported that in 1990 trends for birth defects showed 29 types increasing, 2 decreasing, and 7 unchanged.

Reproductive disorders are also increasing. For instance, ectopic pregnancies (pregnancies that arise outside the uterus) have quadrupled in the last twenty years. The prevalence of endometriosis, a painful disease involving the lining of the uterus, is increasing steadily. And couples are having ever more difficulty conceiving children.

POTENT IMMUNE SYSTEM POISONS

dioxin, a very toxic chemical formed in combustion and pulping of paper

PCBs

cadmium

lead, chromium, copper, nickel, tin, vanadium

mercury

tin compounds— especially organotin

DDT, chlordane, dieldrin, heptachlor, lindane, mirex, toxaphene

pesticides, including carbamates, carbaryl, carbofuran, and malathion

chlorine chemicals used for dry cleaning and formed during water treatment

Chemicals in the Food Chain

How do these poisons get into our systems? In the early 1950s an unlikely discovery changed the way livestock were grown in the United States. Young chickens were given nutrient-rich antibiotic culture waste causing the chickens to grow substantially faster, giving livestock growers more bang for the buck. This culture waste product has now turned into a multimillion-dollar business. Over 50 percent of the antibiotics manufactured in the U.S. today are added directly to the feed of poultry, pigs, and beef cattle. As a dark consequence, it is generally agreed that feeding antibiotics to livestock is causing antibiotic-resistant bacteria to develop and spread. Multiple-antibiotic resistant microbes are becoming widely prevalent in the environment, and drug-resistant bacteria are turning up at hospitals. The massive overuse of antibiotics on livestock is directly responsible for an increase in human infectious diseases.

In recent years food technology has led to sweeping changes in the nutritional composition of diets in the developed world. The agricultural revolution brought profound changes in our ability to produce and store many different foods. Historically there has never before been such a diversity of crops. Yet the diets of the industrialized world remain "wrapped in plastic" and are largely composed of fat and free sugars, or simple carbohydrates. More important, an explosive increase in overprocessed foods has lead to a table menu that has been stripped of essential chemopreventives, the good guys in a diet. Modern prepackaged foods have almost completely lost the substances that help ward off illness.

Is this a brand-new problem? Probably not. Lead poisoning may have caused the fall of the Roman Empire. Both the Greeks and Romans exposed themselves to colossal amounts of lead from food, medicines, water, cooking vessels, and wine. In Rome an elaborate series of cisterns and pipes supplied water. These pipes were made from cast lead sheets. And wine was typically heated and sweetened with sapa, a sugary mixture that had been heated and re-heated in lead vessels. So every time it was heated the sapa became contaminated with more lead. It has been postulated that the high childhood mortality, as well as the low birth rate among the Roman ruling class, may have been due to lead poisoning.

More recently lead has been associated with learning disabilities, such as attention deficit disorder and aggressive behavior. At least seven studies have shown that violent criminals have elevated levels of lead, cadmium, manganese, mercury, and other toxics in their bodies, compared with prisoners who are not violent.

The Achilles' Heel

A central theory holds that chronic degenerative diseases result from a disorder in the mitochondria, the energy sources contained in every cell. The delicate mitochondria are vulnerable for a number of reasons.

The mitochondria, like small but mighty furnaces, produce energy at a constant rate, forming reactive chemicals as a by-product. Since mitochondria generate reactive chemicals, they also take the brunt of their toxicity. To complicate matters, the mitochondria lack a protective covering for their DNA that is found on DNA elsewhere in the cell. They also lack an efficient system for DNA repair.

The structure and function of the mitochondria has remained unchanged over millions of years of evolution. However, in recent years the mitochondria's environment has been radically altered by a number of poisons—aluminum, antibiotics, arsenic, cadmium, lead, manganese, mercury, pesticides, and tin. All can be deadly to the mitochondria. Without mitochondria human life is not possible.

It turns out the mitochondria may be weaker than we thought, and are therefore the key to the modern degenerative illnesses.

Poison sources

So where are pollutants found? How do you get exposed to them? Lead can be found in paint, paint dust, colored newsprint, soil, and water. Rice and vegetables cooked in lead-contaminated water will absorb 80 percent of the lead. Some canned foods contain lead. Lead is found in food wrapping, and sometimes the grinding of meat will increase the lead content. Lead is used in the plastic insulation of wires. It is also lurking in calcium supplements (see appendix D).

Cadmium is typically found in very high amounts in organ meats like liver, and especially kidney. Recently a German study linked the high intake of meat and organ meat (kidney and liver) to increased rates of Parkinson's disease. Shellfish like snails, oysters, mussels, shrimp, and crab, and some fish as well tend to have high amounts of cadmium. Shellfish are exposed to cadmium from the water, then they accumulate it by attaching it to cadmium-binding proteins. Cadmium is also found in cereal grains, root crops, and leafy vegetables. It is more readily taken up by plants than are other metals.

Cadmium is an extremely persistent chemical which progressively accumulates in soft tissues, especially the kidney, and through age it seems to have correlated with the onset of chronic disease. Cadmium can pollute the soil by fallout from the air, or it can come from commercial fertilizers or irrigation water. Cigarettes are another source of cadmium. Smoking one pack a day might double the daily absorbed burden of cadmium.

Mercury is commonly found in fish and seafood, and is easily absorbed through the diet. For this reason we need to limit the amount of seafood we consume, especially fish that prey on other fish. The predatory fish such as shark, swordfish, pike, and barracuda (any fish with teeth) will have much higher levels of mercury and PCBs. So if you eat seafood, select deep ocean halibut and flounder. Stay away from freshwater fish since they tend to have higher amounts of mercury. Mercury is the least persistent of the toxic triad.

Finally, lead dulls IQ, cadmium causes kidney disorders, and mercury causes toxicity to the nervous system. Unfortunately, these effects seem tobe irreversible.

Chapter Recap

- Every year about 1,000 new chemicals are added to a stockpile of 70,000 chemicals used in industry.
- We can now detect over 600 different chemicals in our bodies that were not present before the 1900s.
- A growing number of diseases are related to escalating chemical exposure.
- Reducing pollutants deters the risk of chronic illnesses.
- To fend off a polluted world, humans must adopt a cancer-busting regimen.

Chronic Disease & the Environment

In the last 100 years the number of people with so-called chronic illnesses has soared. The illnesses are called "chronic" because of their relentless, lingering effects. They don't strike overnight; instead they emerge without warning, with subtle symptoms like tiredness or just general blahs. These conditions often cripple people who are older, yet more young people are also succumbing. The symptoms persist, and after a while they change into something that seriously affects the quality of life—something that can finally be called an illness or disease.

> *All substances are poisons; there is none which is not a poison. The right dose differentiates a poison and a remedy.*
> —Paracelsus, 1493–1541

According to the National Cancer Institute, the incidence rate for almost all cancers has steadily increased since the 1950s.

Environmental Illness

A growing number of chronic diseases are related to the environment. Medical researchers believe that increased chemical exposure has resulted in environmental illnesses such as asthma, multiple chemical sensitivity, Parkinson's disease, non-Hodgkin's lymphoma, and aplastic anemia.

ENVIRONMENTAL CAUSES OF CANCER	
ENVIRONMENTAL DISEASES	**SUSPECTED AGENTS**
Asthma	lung irritants
Multiple chemical sensitivity	solvents and smoke
Parkinson's disease	pollutants and pesticides[1]
Non-Hodgkin's lymphoma[2]	herbicides
Aplastic anemia[3]	benzene

[1] Also linked to paper and pulp mill pollutants and manganese exposure
[2] A malignant cancer of the lymph nodes
[3] A deficiency in the production of red blood cells

Immune system disorders such as asthma, diabetes, multiple sclerosis, and lupus are increasing. Asthma is a serious breathing disorder characterized by a narrowing of the airways, making breathing almost impossible. Asthma is on the rise and the underlying cause is not fully understood. But air pollution, cigarette smoke, chemical vapors, and aerosol sprays can trigger asthma attacks. Asthma is especially increasing among children.

Multiple Chemical Sensitivities (MCS)

Recently a new immune disease called *multiple chemical sensitivities (MCS)* has surfaced. MCS is a condition triggered by exposure to certain chemicals and environmental pollutants, and it affects many organ systems. People afflicted with MCS become increasingly sensitive and reactive to low levels of various chemicals that previously did not cause a reaction. Perfume, cigarette smoke, new carpets or paint, and household cleaning products all elicit an adverse reaction at low levels of exposure. The symptoms commonly include disturbances in the respiratory, immune, and gastrointestinal systems. It appears that the incidence of MCS is rising.

Chronic Fatigue Syndrome (CFS)

CFS strikes about 2 million Americans every year. Sufferers complain of being tired all day, yet at night they can't sleep. Why? The syndrome seems to involve a melange of viruses such as herpes (Epstein-Barr), cytomegalovirus, and yeast. The cause of chronic fatigue syndrome has become the million-dollar question.

Nervous System Disorders

Nervous system disorders such as Lou Gehrig's and Parkinson's disease are also increasing. The more common is Parkinson's disease, first described in England in 1817 during the industrial revolution. Before 1817 the disease was virtually unknown. Parkinson sufferers eventually lose voluntary control of their movements, reflected in muscular rigidity and overexaggerated movements.

Studies have linked pesticide use in Quebec, Canada, to increased Parkinson's disease. Recently it has been shown that environmental factors, not genetic factors, cause this debilitating neurologic disease. People who are exposed to pesticides, or who live near pulp and paper mills, have an increased risk of contracting Parkinson's disease.

Learning Disorders

In children, learning disorders are escalating rapidly. Attention deficit disorder (ADD) is characterized by a short attention span, poor memory, and the inability to follow directions. ADD has increased 500 percent in the last forty-five years. A National Research Council study shows evidence that lead exposure 50 percent below the safe level can cause ADD in children. Another learning disorder, autism, was first described in 1938.

Part of the increase in learning disorders is associated with better diagnosis and better understanding of the problems. However, studies show an increased prevalence of learning disorders in children who live near heavily traveled freeways. This highly suggests that part of the problem is originating from the environment.

Endocrine Disrupters

Because we have failed to quickly distinguish the side effects of industrial chemicals, we have been bathing in a sea of estrogen-like compounds. Many items with vastly different chemical structures, from plastics to marijuana, can mimic the female hormone estrogen. It is generally accepted that women with high estrogen levels have a greater risk of cancer in general, and especially breast cancer.

A careful survey of environmental pollutants such as the insecticide DDT, industrial PCBs (polychlorinated biphenyls), and petroleum by-products show that these all possess estrogen activity. PCBs have recently been linked to depressed immune systems, and even to reduced fertility in males. Used extensively in electrical transformers, PCBs are oily liquids that are very stable and do not conduct electricity. PCBs are so stable that they have persisted in our environment and in our food, even though they were banned from production in 1976.

Alzheimer's

Alzheimer's disease is a genetic disease. Recent research tells us that 80 percent of the late-onset type is related to a genetic anomaly. But perhaps the true cause is environmental. There was a time when there was no Alzheimer's disease; it was first described in 1906 by Alois Alzheimer. It is possible that unfortunate people are now susceptible because of a slightly different genetic makeup that predisposes them to the toxic ravages of the twentieth century. Environmental factors may be creating diseases we never would see without the presence of modern pollutants.

The Silence of the Brain

Why do you take the precaution of wearing a helmet when you ride a bicycle or rollerblade? Because, when injured, the brain cannot easily repair itself. Yet every day we silently damage our brain with our food, water, and air. Toxicity to the nervous system is particularly destructive since it cannot regenerate, so all damage is permanent. While brain cells are dying you can't feel the pain; deep inside the brain there are no cells to detect pain! The nervous system is quietly destroyed until the brain's reserve tissue is cut to the point where a functional disorder may arise.

Fortunately, the brain has reserve tissue. You have heard that most people only use 25 percent of their brain capacity. The important point is that the other 75 percent is reserve tissue, and it is just as important as the active tissue. All organs have some reserve capacity. But every decade that we age, we are losing the reserve capacity found in many organ systems. In the brain, for example, you do not see Parkinson's disease until about 70 to 80 percent of a specific neuron (the dopinergic variety) is destroyed. If the rate of destruction is accelerated beyond normal (and who knows what is "normal" in modern times?), Parkinson's disease occurs. The illness expresses itself through loss of motor function, and the victim walks with extreme rigidity, if at all.

Parkinson's disease was the first documented casualty of the industrial revolution. Unfortunately many more illnesses have followed, and more have yet to emerge.

Chemophobia

It's not surprising in today's world when patience starts wearing thin. Every day the media bombards us with discovery of yet another food item or environmental agent that causes cancer. Books classifying the poisons in our environment are being published at an alarming rate. There is a flood of seemingly conflicting information concerning cancer. People are throwing their hands in the air. Why bother? As far as the average person is concerned, everything causes cancer! The truth is, not everything is linked to cancer, and many foods and substances actually prevent cancer! But the truth is useless unless you can apply it to your everyday life. Let's take a moment to examine a central principle at the heart of the science of toxicology, and look at the naturally toxic agents in your diet.

In general, the most abundant substances in the earth's crust, such as sand or silica, are less toxic than rare elements. Metal-like compounds, such as selenium, are found in small amounts in the earth's crust, so they are rare. Since life has evolved in a naturally occurring blend of chemicals and elements, we have developed means to tolerate the most abundant chemicals. Selenium is toxic, but it is a necessary element for proper nutrition (in extremely small amounts, around 1 millionth of a gram). Iodine causes thyroid cancer when you ingest it in excess, but it also causes cancer when you don't have enough.

The vast majority of people believe that if some is good, then more is better. In some cases this might be true, but only to a point. The devil is in the dose. One central concept of toxicology is the dose/response relationship. In a toxicologist's world everything is viewed as a poison. Water is one of the most convincing examples, since it is believed by many to be nontoxic, yet it can be fatal if taken down the windpipe.

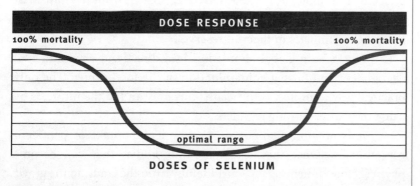

DOSE RESPONSE

100% mortality   100% mortality

optimal range

DOSES OF SELENIUM

Figure 5

Avoiding Overdose

High levels of dietary selenium have been associated with decreased risk of digestive system cancer. It would seem to make sense that increased doses of selenium will provide more protection. The "more is better" logic can get one into toxic trouble quickly. The safeguards hinge on a protective system that uses selenium as a cofactor in order to be active. There are only so many selenium molecules that can be used; once the system is saturated, no more protection will be offered, and in fact, further increases will risk toxicity.

As a result of this narrow window of protective benefits, it is important not to oversupplement yourself with anticancer agents. A morsel of cancer-cutting agent taken regularly every day is much more effective than a massive amount consumed all at once. Aristotle's truism "Everything in moderation" is certainly applicable to the dose/response relationship.

If a chemical becomes toxic, it may simply boil down to how much gets in and how much goes out. If more goes in than comes out, there is an internal stockpile, so toxicity and illness can result. In the case of many environmental pollutants, 95 percent can be absorbed, with very few being eliminated. A small amount in the daily diet can, over time, result in a level that leads to illness.

Avoiding Toxic Chemicals

We all have some kind of environmental pollution stored in our bodies; regrettable as it may seem, chemical pollution is global. Even penguins in remote areas like Antarctica, isolated from the industrial world by thousands of miles, have an impressive number of environmental contaminates in their fat reserves.

Increases in global population lead directly to environmental degradation and further contamination of the food supply. The only practical way to protect your health, currently and in the future, is by using the cancer-busting regimen.

It is of utmost importance to limit our intake of persistent contaminates. Once they cross into our bodies they can become physical embodiments and persist literally from the cradle to the grave. These persistent poisons include the toxic metal triad of cadmium, lead, and to a lesser extent mercury and the so-called organo-chlorine chemicals like PCB and DDT.

The shocking thing is these chemicals have no function in our body except to poison it. Many have been produced by a mad scramble of industrial activities, and were not so available before 200 years ago. Studies suggest that many poisons may exert toxic effects never dreamed of. They can zap energy, play havoc with the immune system, form major cancers, and cause nervous system disorders. Beneath the layers of controversy about chemical-related illnesses, the toxic triad appears again and again in the heated debates.

What is the evidence? How are they so persistent?

By most reckonings, lead in the diet is not well absorbed. Adults absorb 5 to 15 percent. Children, on the other hand, can absorb over 40 percent. But once absorbed, lead stays around for an extremely long time—twenty, thirty, even forty years and longer.

Cadmium is not well absorbed from dietary sources either (5 to 8 percent remains in the body). But once it enters your system, it can become a lifetime molecular mate, staying around well over thirty years. Cadmium is associated with increased respiratory and prostate cancers.

In contrast, mercury, which is found primarily in fish and other seafood, is very well absorbed, at greater than 90 percent. Mercury does reside for a shorter time than lead or cadmium. But it's alarming that a diet rich in mercury can quickly build to levels that will cause toxicity.

Chapter Recap

- Many chemical agents in the environment may cause cancer.
- The only practical way to protect your health is by using the cancer-busting regimen.

Protecting Yourself Against a Polluted Planet

Can you imagine a world free of heart disease and cancer? Can you imagine a place where osteoporosis, stroke, diabetes, and Parkinson's disease are virtually unknown? Could this be the United States 100 years from now? No, it is reality today in the less developed countries of the world! The nonindustrialized countries have successfully avoided heart disease, cancer, and stroke, the so-called diseases of affluence. In the industrialized world, pestilence and famine are relics of the past; but the chronic illnesses of heart disease, cancer, and stroke have taken their places, becoming formidable and feared.

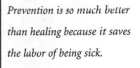

Prevention is so much better than healing because it saves the labor of being sick.

—Thomas Adams,
seventeenth-century physician

The affluent diet that is so rich and seemingly varied is in fact severely deficient. Over 90 percent of Americans do not eat enough foods that can prevent disease. The biggest health risk we face is concealed in our food. Your diet can magnify your risk of disease, or it can alleviate it.

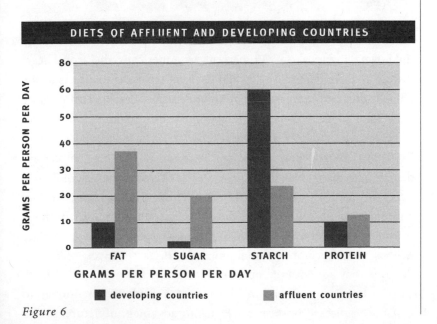

Figure 6

For millennia humans have consumed massive amounts of plants with their indigestible fiber. In fact the digestive system of humans evolved around the intake of high amounts of dietary plant fiber. In the last three centuries, however, Western or affluent diets have progressively refined and removed complex carbohydrates or fiber, increasing fat and sugar levels instead. On the scale of human evolution, these are radical changes to our food supply.

DIETARY CAUSES OF CANCER			
	FAT	ALCOHOL	SMOKED, SALTY FOODS	EXCESS BODY WEIGHT
Mouth	●	●		
Throat		●	●	
Breast	●	●		●
Stomach			●	
Colon	●			
Rectum	●	●		
Liver		●	●	
Uterus				●
Prostate	●			

Before the 1920s, coronary heart disease was virtually unknown. Today about 40 percent of Americans die from heart disease. A mere decade or two ago the long-term health effects of the affluent diet surfaced, and this way of eating is clearly causing more harm than good. It has become the prime culprit in our spiraling rates of heart disease, cancer, and stroke.

Our biggest health risk can be found in the fact that certain dietary ingredients may increase, as well as decrease, the risk of illness. Recently one of the most spectacular scientific findings has been that anticancer agents are found in the ordinary foods humans have been consuming for centuries. Many of these guardians against cancer are neither vitamins nor essential minerals. In fact, as you will soon discover, they are not even nutrients!

It turns out that we don't need a medical practitioner to marshal defenses against cancer. By taking advantage of natural cancer guardians—that is, by preparing our meals correctly and eating the right foods (the chemopreventive foods that contain cancer-busting agents)—we can ward off cancer, heart disease, stroke, and other chronic illnesses.

The majority of chemopreventive agents can be classified into three categories: *inhibitors, blocking agents,* and *suppressing agents.* Most chemopreventive agents don't work in mysterious ways; they simply block a toxic process or hinder the formation of cancer-producing chemicals. In some cases they conquer cancer by counteracting the toxic event that causes a precancerous tumor, or they suppress the cancer response. Still other chemopreventive agents, such as selenium, augment a normal bodily defense system.

Each chemopreventive food group operates in different and often perplexing ways. It's going to take researchers a long time to sift through results. Scientists still have not unraveled all the mysteries of cancer, but as time goes on there is increased understanding of its workings.

Flavonoids

Flavonoids are a family of over 4,000 naturally occurring plant compounds that include polyphenols. In order to unlock the secret to how polyphenols work, scientists have been looking at how they combat the toxic transformations of oxygen.

Contrary to general belief oxygen is highly toxic and reacts with many substances, triggering them to become *oxidized,* or chemically altered, like the rust on exposed metals. Polyphenols act like antioxidants, or *rustproofing agents,* that are believed to hasten the oxidation of cholesterol, thus protecting against heart disease. Compelling evidence suggests that oxidized cholesterol is a prime villain in creation of artery-clogging plaque, which plays a critical role in heart disease.

Chocolate

Thanks to flavonoids, it may be that chocolate is part of a healthful diet. Cocoa was discovered in the 1500s following one of Columbus's voyages to the New World. This may always be controversial, but recent studies show that the flavonoids in chocolate protect from heart disease. These flavonoids lower the risk of heart disease by acting as antioxidants, preventing fat (or LDL—low-density lipoprotein) in the blood from oxidizing and clogging the arteries. Cocoa flavonoids naturally keep the butter fat in chocolate from turning rancid. These preservative traits of cocoa, along with its merits as a sustained energy source (due to its high-fat content), have not gone unnoticed. During World War II, American soldiers in heavy combat were often rationed three chocolate bars each day as their only source of food.

Dark or semisweet chocolate is the best form because it contains more flavonoids. But before you go wild eating chocolate, recall that Aristotle said, "Everything in moderation." Too much wine or too much chocolate will throw your body out of balance. If you snack on chocolate, try to find dark types that contain 70 percent cocoa, and make sure that sugar or butter fat is not the first ingredient listed.

Polyphenols

Polyphenols are present in many foods, including green tea, black tea, licorice, and spices. Remarkably, white wine and processed grape juice will not usually provide protection since polyphenols are mostly present in red wine, and they are destroyed by the heat during processing of grape juice. However, grape skins are a major source of polyphenols and may boost athletic performance as well.

Garlic

Historically, garlic has had a formidable reputation as a dewormer, aphrodisiac, and vampire repellent. More recently, garlic is believed to prevent the common cold and flu. Now scientists are looking beyond folklore to demonstrate that garlic deters cancer and heart disease. When garlic is crushed or cooked it releases more than seventy different sulfur-bearing compounds. These compounds impart the distinct garlic odor, and they possess anticancer properties. Recent studies indicate that garlic lowers cholesterol, hinders cancer cell growth, and has antiviral and antifungal properties. However, odorless garlic pills are not likely to provide complete medicinal benefits.

Olive Oil

Experiments with olive oil have shown that it, too, is biologically friendly. Monounsaturated fats occurring in olives and macadamia nuts can ameliorate heart disease. Olive oil has long been a staple of the Mediterranean diet and current studies have linked it to decreased heart disease on the islands of Corfu and Crete.

Heart Disease Prevention Meal Plan

Rely on These:

- Antioxidants (vitamins A, C, E, and beta carotene)
- B vitamins (vitamins B12, B6, folic acid, biotin, niacin)
- Trace minerals (selenium, copper, zinc, magnesium, manganese)
- Foods (fresh fruits and vegetables, red wine, dark grapes, green tea—high in antioxidants and manganese—garlic, high-fiber foods, chocolate flavonoids, monounsaturated fats such as olive, sesame, and canola oil, fish oils rich in omega-3 fats, brazil nuts, almonds, pecans, and walnuts)
- Miscellaneous (enteric-coated aspirin—one every other day)

Avoid:

- High-fat diet
- Animal products (dairy products, poultry, meats)
- High-iron foods like red meat
- Trans-fatty acids found in margarine and other products that include partially hydrogenated vegetable oils
- Fried foods (oxidized fats and cholesterol are known to cause heart disease)
- Cigarette smoking and tobacco
- Elevated blood lipoproteins (cholesterol), increased blood pressure, elevated sugar levels—all risk factors for heart disease

Tomatoes
Scientists have also shown that tomatoes suppress the formation of cancer-producing chemicals. The tomato contains vitamin C and the retinoid lycopene, both of which are believed to forestall the formation of cancer-inciting chemicals.

Whole Foods

Dozens of studies have endowed spices (such as rosemary and sage), soybeans, grapefruit juice, licorice, cauliflower, brussels sprouts, broccoli, and citrus fruits and oils as superior cancer bashers. To remain healthy, rely on whole foods (since many chemopreventive agents are destroyed by heat or food-processing techniques) in conjunction with vitamin supplements.

Vitamins and Nutrients

Many vitamins and other nutrients are also chemopreventive: beta-carotene, minerals such as zinc and calcium, fish oils such as omega-3 fats, and nondigestible fibers. Pharmaceutical companies are also developing synthetic drugs reputed to be chemopreventive, including retinoid derivatives and various compounds.

Healthful Benefits of Fiber

Fiber inhibits intestinal tumors. Coarse fiber that does not dissolve and form a gel or insoluble fiber is more consistent in blocking cancer.

THE SCOOP ON FIBER

binds up toxic bile acids—
fiber binds up bile acids and facilitates their removal

dilutes the intestinal contents

reduces the formation of more toxic secondary bile acids

Fiber reduces passage time in the gut. The faster gut contents are expelled, the less contact time, the less conversion of toxic secondary bile acids occurs and less damage to bowel surfaces.

Those who eat fiber often don't realize there are two general classes of dietary fiber: soluble and insoluble. Soluble fiber will dissolve in water and form a gel-like substance. Soluble fiber is found in apples, grapefruit, and grains like oat and psyllium. In contrast, insoluble fiber undergoes minimal change in the intestine and is passed out mostly unchanged. Insoluble fibers include bran cereals, whole wheat, and rice bran.

The physical and chemical form of fiber is important; finely ground fiber is less effective then coarse fiber. Fibers that are poorly fermented by bacteria (like cellulose, which is a common plant fiber, and corn bran) increase the fecal weight more than fibers that are easily fermented.

Dietary fiber also plays a role with the bacteria that populate the intestinal tract. These bacteria are central to the handling of chemicals passing through the intestines. Since the gut is estimated to house 400 to 500 species of bacteria, the bacteria that line the intestines can profoundly influence the toxicity of ingested chemicals. The bacteria can cause you to absorb more, and they can make them more toxic. The large intestine is the most heavily populated area of the intestine. Unabsorbed food may play an important role in providing specific nutrients to microbes. And this is probably why environmental chemicals—when they pass into the intestine—are also metabolized by the gut bacteria. High-fiber diets speed the removal, and they lessen the bacterial conversion of environmental contaminates.

Mercury is significantly recycled in bile, then is reabsorbed by the gut. Wheat bran not only reduces the uptake of mercury by 30 percent, but it also removes mercury from the body up to 43 percent faster.

A recent study has shown that the environmental chemical PCB can be bound by rice bran fiber and by spinach fibers. The encouraging news is that rice and spinach fiber cause a tremendous increase in PCB excretion. Fibers *not* effective in binding PCB are burdock (popular in Asian food), cabbage, soybean, radish, carrot, corn, and cellulose.

To remove pollutants, drink plenty of water (which increases chemical removal through urine). Also include fiber from the following foods in your diet every day:

- Wheat bran (binds cadmium and mercury)
- Rice bran, spinach (binds PCB)
- Psyllium, oat bran (increases bile removal)

Zapping Cancer

Certainly everyone should practice chemoprevention, especially people who have a high risk of cancer and heart disease. If you are exposed to carcinogens at work, cigarette smoke, alcohol, or excess sun, your health will benefit from a constant infusion of cancer-zapping agents.

Research makes it clear that there is no single magic concoction that can protect us from all forms of cancer. Be very skeptical about inflated health claims based on one *miracle nutrient* (see appendix B).

COMPOUNDS THAT REVERSE CANCER PROGRESS

soybeans—diadzein

vitamin D

butyric acid—formed from bacteria's action on dietary fiber

vitamin A

beta carotene

fish oil—DHA

Chemopreventives have been proven to work together, and independently, by providing unique forms of protection not duplicated by other food groups. Chemopreventive food groups consumed along with anticancer vitamins and minerals will provide you with the most cancer-busting potential.

Chemoprevention

Traditionally the focus of medicine has been intervention, not prevention. Emphasis has been on identifying cancer-producing chemicals or *carcinogens*, as well as on developing more sensitive cancer detection methods. But there is a simpler solution: stopping cancer cell growth before it becomes lethal.

In 1982 the National Cancer Institute established a Chemoprevention Branch, with the mission of developing chemopreventive drugs, nutrients, minerals, and non-nutritive compounds.

AIMS OF CHEMOPREVENTION

preserve the integrity of DNA

prevent mutation (alteration) of DNA

enhance DNA repair systems

prevent promotion of cancer cells

prevent toxicity to tissues

enhance detoxification and removal systems

enhance favorable hormones

enhance favorable bacteria in the intestine

It turns out that prevention also includes identifying certain foods and agents that should be avoided. Chemoprevention interrupts the processes of cancer or chronic disease by presenting stumbling blocks that inhibit the growth of the disease, or that even reverse the disease process.

Chemoprevention squashes or reverses the number of cells on their way to cancer, or in other words, it intervenes with initiated cells by deterring their promotion. Cancer-thwarting agents cause promoted cells to regain control of their own division, thereby reversing or inhibiting promotion of cancer cells. Cancer-suppressing agents may also augment natural defense systems, antioxidant enzymes, and DNA repair enzymes. Ultimately the science of chemoprevention attempts to protect the integrity of DNA, which is the master blueprint all cells follow.

As a formidable antagonist to cancer and heart disease, chemoprevention is making use of cancer-slashing substances such as drugs and agents found naturally in red wine, green tea, cabbage, tomatoes, garlic, and even fish oils. If you follow a chemopreventive lifestyle, you could potentially nullify your risk of cancer by upwards of 80 percent.

Some scientists have estimated even higher risk reduction, while others have issued conservative estimates near 40 percent. In either case, we are talking about significant reductions in the risk of contracting either cancer or heart disease. By retarding your cancer risk you also gain protection from heart disease, since heart disease and cancer share similar causes. In addition, there is growing evidence that chemopreventive mixtures can intercede in the toxicity of environmental agents such as ultraviolet light, tobacco smoke, and chemical pollution. Clearly, the new directive should be the search for, and discovery of, new substances that block cancer and chronic illness.

Chemopreventive agents can be either natural or synthetic. Nature provides an extensive menu of chemopreventive agents found naturally in fruits, vegetables, tea, spices, and herbs. Fresh fruits and vegetables are rich sources of vitamins and other non-nutritives (some of which are not yet identified, and others that may never be), and have proven to be powerful in suppressing the rates of most cancers.

Proteins

A chemopreventive diet may require not only the addition of certain foods to your menu but the subtraction of others. Some of the things you should think about eliminating in part or entirely are things you once thought were good for you.

It is known that the source or type of protein influences metal uptake. In experiments with dietary protein given to animals, casein (a milk protein) has been shown to result in higher lead levels in the brain, liver, and kidney, compared to animals who received their protein from a soybean diet. A diet supplemented with soybean meal reduces lead absorption and toxicity. On the other hand, it is believed that the fat content in milk enhances absorption. When the amount of dietary fat given to animals is increased from 5 to 20 percent, the level of lead in the blood doubles. The type of fat is also important. Saturated butterfat causes the greatest increase, whereas polyunsaturated sunflower oils have little effect on lead uptake. The milk sugar lactose also shows an enhanced absorption of lead compared to other dietary sugars, while the fruit sugar pectin is found to bind up lead, decreasing its absorption.

Meat

For millennia domesticated animals have provided humans with a good source of protein through meat and meat products. However, with changing farming practices and increasing industrialization, meat, poultry, fish, and dairy products now account for between 60 and 80 percent of the pesticide and organo-chlorine chemical residues in the American diet. Organo-chlorine chemicals are a family of industrial chemicals that have become widespread in our environment. A number of these chemicals like PCB and dioxin have been shown to be potent immune system poisons. Of the pesticide residues, only about 10 percent come from vegetables, fruits, and grains. So even if you consume only commercial rather than organic produce, if you limit your meat, fish, dairy, and poultry intake, you can partially avoid this pesticide and industrial chemical burden.

The Bad News About Meat

- High fat
- Protein overload (excess protein is linked to other diseases)
- Sodium overload (meat is high in sodium)
- Iron overload (iron from meat is easily absorbed and can cause heart disease and cancer)
- Contains immune system poisons, such as dioxin and PCB
- Contains arachidonic acid that is turned into prostaglandins which are linked with cancer
- Contains hormones and antibiotics (drug-resistant bacterial infections are on the rise)
- White blood cell count rises, fat saturates the blood, and sex hormones increase in the body when an oversized portion of meat is eaten

Eating too much red meat can also lead to high iron storage and may increase cancer, as well as heart disease, risk. The type of iron found in red meat is absorbed quite well. Men have only one good mechanism to remove excess iron—by donating blood. On the other hand, women in their reproductive years shed iron monthly. This is one reason men may be more prone to heart disease than women. However, this comparison holds only when women are in their reproductive years. Women in menopause have the same risk of heart disease as men. A recent study in Sweden showed a reduction in cancer risk in blood donors.

How Much Do You Need?

What are our protein requirements? Probably a lot less than originally thought. The protein content of mother's milk would seem to provide a rough gauge of an individual's maximum requirements. After all, infancy is the most nutritionally demanding period in our lives. Rat milk, for instance, is 49 percent protein. Cow's milk is 15 percent protein. It is interesting that human breast milk is only 5 percent protein. Apparently humans have a much smaller protein requirement, even during this intensive growth phase, than many other animals.

The original studies conducted for determining protein requirements in humans were based on rodents, since it is unethical to use humans in studies that would deprive them of protein until diseases appeared. For that reason everyone relied on these old studies, which suggested we need enormous amounts of protein for health. To this day dairy producers perpetuate outdated, false claims for consuming three glasses of milk per day, and meat producers extol the benefits of a meat-based diet. The truth is, there are no health advantages to eating more protein than is required. In fact excess protein is associated with osteoporosis, kidney disease, and cancer.

If you do eat oversized portions of meat, then take the following precautions:

- Check your blood iron regularly.
- Donate blood if your blood iron is high.
- Do not take iron supplements.
- Eat plenty of dark green leafy vegetables.
- Try to consume free-range beef.
- Follow the cancer-busting regimen.

Dairy

When asked what single change in the American diet would produce the greatest health benefits, Washington, D.C.-based pediatrician Dr. Russell Bunai said, "Eliminate dairy products." Besides higher levels of fat, diary products have some serious health effects.

Dangers of Dairy

- Diabetes. Infants with milk allergies make antibodies against milk proteins that are linked to destroying cells in the pancreas.
- Cataracts. The milk sugar galactose builds up in the lens of the eye, causing an irreversible clouding or cataract.
- Increased risk of ovarian cancer. Dairy, especially from cows treated with hormones, is linked to ovarian cancer and to elevated breast and prostate cancer.
- Increased intake of environmental chemicals.
- Increased heart disease.
- Increased lead, cadmium, and mercury uptake and toxicity. (Milk enhances the uptake of lead, cadmium, mercury, and other metals.)
- Increased salmonella infections. (The Center for Disease Control has warned elderly or pregnant women not to eat soft cheese or drink milk.)
- Increased digestive disorders in infants. (Many infants show colic problems due to cow's milk.)
- Lactose intolerance. (As people get older they normally lose the ability to digest lactose, forming gas in the intestine, bloating, cramps, and diarrhea.)

Don't Panic—Eat Organic!

Is it better to eat organic produce than commercial produce? You bet it is! The major difference lies in the use of pesticides and commercial fertilizers. Commercially grown fruits and vegetables have more pesticide residues than organic varieties. Also, compounds like nitrates (which can be converted into cancer-producing chemicals) are more prevalent in commercially grown produce.

Ten Ways to Reduce Pollutant Loads

Eat less meat, dairy, seafood, fish, and poultry.

- If you eat meat, get free-range[1] beef, chicken, turkey, and eggs (see appendix F).
- Eat more organic vegetables and fruit (see appendix F).
- Get off the pesticide treadmill (see appendix C).
- Peel or wash commercial produce (see appendix F).
- Eat more fiber.
- Drink more purified water.
- Don't drink any tap water or beverages made with tap water
- Don't use aluminum and plastic in cooking (see appendix E).
- Make sure your home is lead-free.

Organic produce will generally contain higher amounts of essential minerals because of crop rotation. Commercially grown crops are often not rotated in different soils, but are grown over and over in the same mineral-depleted soils. This is why extensive use of fertilizers is required for these crops. Organically grown produce has been shown to have up to three times more minerals and trace elements than commercial produce.

Studies also show that beneficent plant chemicals called *phytochemicals* are higher in organic produce. Many of these phytochemicals have been linked to reduced cancer risk. Beyond this, organically grown produce has a much better taste!

Healthy Reasons to Eat Organic

- Fewer herbicide residues
- Fewer insecticide residues
- Fewer fungicide residues
- Fewer toxic metals
- Fewer toxic nitrates
- Many more essential and trace minerals
- No hormones (organic cows are not given hormones to increase milk production)

---

[1] Free-range refers to meat, poultry, and eggs produced with the freedom of the range, and animals not given hormones or growth stimulants.

- No antibiotics (organically raised animals are not given lifelong antibiotics)
- More healthful agents (organic grapes, for example, contain more resveratrol, a heart protective agent)
- Tastes much better and you can eat the skin

To repeat: Diet is the most common source of persistent chemicals. Preventing toxic exposure is your paramount objective. Because of widespread cadmium, lead, and mercury contamination, limit your daily intake of seafood, such as oysters, mussels, snails, fish, shrimp, and crab; also limit processed foods and commercially grown produce. Never eat organ meats like liver and kidney. Avoid canned foods. Get a daily supply of:

- Vitamin C
- Calcium
- Zinc
- Selenium
- Sulfur amino acids (cysteine, methionine)
- Essential fats (soybeans or walnuts)

Foods that are high in calcium include oranges, spinach, rhubarb, collards, dried figs, turnips, kale, okra, tofu (or soybeans), white and pinto beans, broccoli, and baked beans

Precautions

Be careful with supplements. Some zinc supplements are contaminated with cadmium. Also, cadmium is absorbed from drinking water more than from other dietary sources. On the other hand, plant products like lignan and cellulose dramatically reduce cadmium absorption into the body. Also, calcium supplements in the form of bone meal may be contaminated with lead. Be aware that infants and children absorb more metals, especially lead. So don't use milk to supplement calcium in the diet because milk tends to increase lead and cadmium (and other heavy metal) absorption.

Detoxing the Body

How do we enhance the removal of environmental chemicals from the body? The liver processes most of the normal dietary components, and it also facilitates removal of environmental chemicals. One goal of the liver is to alter chemicals with long resident times, such as benzene, into compounds that will dissolve in water and get passed into the urine. However, the liver can bungle the removal attempt and in fact can actually activate some nontoxic substances so that they become toxic ones. Benzene is a good example of a chemical that can be activated to a carcinogen by normal liver functions.

The kidney provides another critical removal system. The kidney filters the blood; in an average person, about 180 liters of fluid are filtered each day. Compounds that are small tend to be excreted in urine and eliminated by the kidneys. Adequate water and fluid intake is vital for the continued removal of a large number of foreign chemicals (such as penicillin). By drinking enough water and properly irrigating your kidneys, you remove many foreign chemicals before they build up to toxic amounts.

Therefore you do have some control over the balance between how much of a substance goes in, how much becomes stored, and how much is removed. When the scales tip toward storage, troublesome reactions can take place. There are many avenues through which environmental agents can enter your body, but most do so through your mouth. You can inhale others. Yet there are only two main avenues out of the body—urine and feces.

In order to understand the behavior of compounds that are fatlike and tend to be stored in fat deposits (where they may persist for years), remember that oil and water do not mix. A common example is salad dressing. The oil (or fat) will not stay mixed with the vinegar, which behaves similarly to water. Normally our liver transforms fatlike chemicals into ones that will dissolve in water, so then they can be passed into urine.

Bile dissolves fat. Bile is a dark green material, which is produced and excreted from the liver. A large high-fat meal will trigger the release of bile, which then acts like a detergent, allowing fats to be dissolved and taken up by the intestine. In order to speed removal, the liver attaches various proteins and sugars to chemicals that have a predilection for bile. Compounds found in broccoli, cauliflower, cabbage, and other plants can increase the activity of these so-called phase II enzymes, and can also increase the removal of compounds into the bile. Some compounds excreted in bile include: arsenic, cadmium, lead, manganese, mercury, and environmental chemicals like DDT and PCBs. Bile is also an extremely important avenue for environmental chemicals that are processed, then excreted, from the liver (biliary secretion). But not everything that is excreted by the bile is removed. Many compounds are cleaved by intestinal bacteria and taken back into the body. The toxic agent goes out of the liver in the bile, and some are passed out of the system altogether; however, intestinal bacteria will unfortunately convert some bile back into the original or an even more toxic form (secondary bile acids), then reabsorb it. The consequence is a vicious cycle of removal and uptake. Removal and re-uptake is the crux of chemical persistence.

That's where the importance of fiber comes in. Fiber binds up the bile and takes it completely out of your system! An increased removal of bile can decrease the uptake and toxicity of environmental chemicals. Toxic chemicals can become permanent fixtures within your own body, or they can be flushed down the toilet.

Chapter Recap

- A Western or affluent diet is severely deficient in cancer-preventing agents.
- If we eat the right foods—foods that contain chemopreventive agents—we can ward off cancer, heart disease, and stroke.
- Chocolate and red wine can be part of a healthful diet.
- Your diet can modify the behavior of pollutants and remove them from your system.
- It's a good idea to limit animal and dairy products.

Other Dietary Traditions

It seems reasonable to assume that if cancer-stifling foods are the staples of the healthy, then people who routinely consume these foods are more likely to live longer. Unprecedented proof lies with two independent populations: Seventh Day Adventists and the Japanese.

Tell me what you eat and I will tell you what you are.

—Anthelme Brillat-Savarin, 1755–1826

Seventh Day Adventists have religious beliefs calling for them to eat five servings of fruits and vegetables every day. On the average, their life span is seven years longer than other Americans.

The Japanese on the average live to almost 80 years, having the longest average life span in the world. Even more astonishing: though Japan has one of the highest per capita rates of cigarette consumption, it has the world's lowest rates of lung cancer! How can this be possible? This data must lead to the conclusion that factors other than cigarettes are involved with the development of lung cancer. What cannot be overlooked is the Japanese diet, which is packed with cancer-busting substances.

Many Japanese and Chinese foods are eaten without cooking, and when they are cooked the process is brief. Freshness is highly prized, so food is eaten as soon as possible after harvesting, usually within minutes. The Japanese make daily expeditions to the market for fresh groceries. They also eat few dairy products and very little red meat.

In contrast, Western diets are prepared with extensive, often high-temperature cooking methods. Americans eat relatively few fresh foods while overconsuming highly processed ones. A typical American family may visit the market once a week and consume meat and dairy products daily.

Western-style cooking generates more cancer-causing agents than were present in the food before it was cooked. And fresh foods like vegetables and fruits, which protect from cancer, have been replaced in Western diets with prepackaged, processed foods with long shelf lives.

Japanese Cuisine

A unique food culture has evolved in Japan due to its mild climate and religious beliefs. The traditional diet consists of a variety of raw food staples such as sushi, seaweed, and rice, as well as many fermented products like soy sauce, miso, natto, tempeh, sake, and salty pickles.

But not every food in the Japanese diet is chemopreventive. Heavily salted raw fish and pickled foods have put the Japanese at high risk for cancers of the stomach.

The Japanese were originally influenced by the Chinese belief that daily diet controls health, disease, and aging. So the Japanese have traditionally used foods with medicinal qualities such as green tea, sesame seeds and oil, sake, rice vinegar, shiitake mushrooms, and various seafoods. Since ancient times it has been believed that tea keeps the mind and soul in a healthy condition. Now pioneering research from Shanghai, China, has established that green tea guards against throat (esophagus) cancer. Further studies confirm that tea dramatically thwarts heart and respiratory disease, and hinders development of prostate cancer as well (discussed in Chapter 10).

Many foods from the traditional Japanese diet, including seaweed and algae (such as the edible brown algae), have shown significant cancer-busting properties. This is partly due to antioxidants that are surprisingly superior to vitamin E and are contained in sesame seeds and *azuki* or red beans. Sesame seeds and sesame oil, which are considered to boost energy and slow aging, are crucial in the Japanese diet. Recently, several new antioxidants were discovered in sesame oil.

Another Japanese staple with legendary powers is the lotus plant and its seeds, which are rich in vitamin E and other antioxidants. For a long time the fermented products of soybeans, such as miso, natto, and tempeh, have been recognized for their significant antioxidant properties.

So it's no wonder the Japanese enjoy such long lives. Their diet is decidedly chemopreventive.

The French Diet

One thing we all know is that diets high in saturated fats and choles-terol are associated with increased risk of heart disease. It is fascinating to note, however, that the French eat almost four times as much butter and three times as much lard as do Americans. The French have higher blood pressure and cholesterol levels. Yet Americans have two and one-half times greater risk of death from heart disease than the French. Crazy as it seems, recent statistics plainly show that the French are nearly three times less likely to develop heart disease than Americans.

Just how do the French manage to avoid cardiac problems? Apparently fat is not the most important dietary item when it comes to heart disease. The French drink very little milk, enjoy large portions of fresh vegetables and fruit, and drink wine with most meals. In fact the average French person drinks nine times as much wine as an American. So it now seems that red wine, a French cultural necessity, has a direct bearing on slashing heart disease. Red wine is one of the most recent substances linked to the chemoprevention of heart disease!

It is now believed that the blood-thinning *resveratrol*, as well as the so-called flavonoids in red wine, are partial antidotes and help maintain a healthy heart. Resveratrol is a natural fungicide produced by grapes and is primarily found in their skins. Because resveratrol is produced in much higher quantities in grapes that are organically grown, organic red grapes may be a good option if you don't want to drink wine. Wine grapes are crushed with the seeds and cluster stems as part of the wine. Grape seeds are also rich sources of the heart-protecting flavonoids, found especially in red wines like pinot noir. While grapes are seasonal, wine can be enjoyed year around.

People from the Mediterranean areas of Europe have reaped benefits from their diet for centuries. It contains three basic cancer-smothering components: red wine, olive oil, and garlic.

Health Benefits of Red Wine

- Thins the blood (red wine reduces platelet activity, which plays a key role in heart attacks)
- May reduce strokes (platelet activity is also related to strokes)

- Contains antioxidants (two glasses boost antioxidant flavonoids by 40 percent)
- Lowers cholesterol (resveratrol in grapes lowers cholesterol)
- Enhances blood flow (red wine causes the blood vessels to relax, promoting a healthy cardiac system)
- Promotes a favorable fat profile (red wine—not white wine—elevates the heart-friendly HDLs)
- May reverse heart disease (blood vessel lesions have been reduced in rabbits fed high cholesterol and red wine)
- May help people with diabetes (alcohol is known to enhance insulin release, which may also be protective in heart disease)
- Blocks LDL oxidation (red wine blocks the oxidation of LDL, a known risk factor in heart disease)
- May prevent tumors (a decreased risk of breast cancer has been shown with wine, while increased risk occurs with beer and liquor)
- May lower the risk of blindness (red wine lowers the risk of macular degeneration in the elderly; beer and liquor do not protect)

Chapter Recap

- Antioxidants in Japanese cuisine reduce cancer risk.
- Resveratrol and flavonoids in the French diet reduce the risk of cancer and heart disease.

The Super Eight Food Groups:
A Diet to Defeat Cancer

More than 2,000 years ago Hippocrates, a Greek physician known as the Father of Medicine, realized the vital link between diet and disease. It's astonishing to the point of regret that it has taken over two millennia for Western medicine to seriously investigate how diet can be a deterrent to disease.

Your food shall be your remedy. Let food be your medicine and let medicine be your food.

—Hippocrates, Greek Physician, 5th Century B.C.

Nutrition with its long and storied history has gone through a series of revolutions. One striking example is the discovery of vitamin C with its link to the disease called scurvy, a disease marked by bleeding, anemia, tooth loss, fetid breath, and gum ulcers. Scurvy plagued generations of adventurers, including the California gold miners, sailors on extended voyages, and others on long ventures without fresh foods. An impressive example of the torment scurvy could inflict was found aboard a Spanish galleon discovered in 1577 adrift in the Sargasso Sea, with the entire crew dead from scurvy.

In Britain it was eventually discovered that scurvy could be halted by consuming a seashore plant called scurvy grass (which explains how the disease was named). Later the British navy replaced scurvy grass with limes and lime juice; henceforth British sailors became known as *limeys*.

To medical researchers the discovery of vitamins, along with their absolute necessity to health, was one of the great scientific achievements of the 20th century. Vitamins in the classic sense are vital factors for sustaining life. A diet lacking a single vitamin or essential mineral will result in disease and eventually death. Vitamins (discussed in detail in chapter 7) paved the way for better health through nutrition, at the same time combating nutrition-related diseases and suffering. During the early years of the vitamin revolution, the entire focus was on taking in sufficient vitamins and minerals to stave off deficiency diseases. The science of nutrition became a trifle boring in 1940 after most vitamins had been discovered. However, there is much more to health than vitamins.

You Call That Food?

In the years following the Second World War, the burgeoning American food industry offered hungry people convenience foods. Heat-and-eat TV dinners, gratefully accepted in busy households, became a national pastime. The average time to shop for and prepare dinner in 1950 was an arduous two and a half hours, compared to a mere seven minutes in 1996. Unfortunately the era of carefree meal preparation has escalated the incidence of cancer and chronic disease.

The modern food industry centers its efforts on processing food by mashing and grinding it, and then caking, baking, toasting, roasting, pasteurizing, sterilizing, and evaporating it until what is left is a meal stripped clean of protective agents. They then add a medley of stabilizing agents, flavor enhancers, thickeners, leavening agents, emulsifiers, humectants, sweeteners, preservatives, and coloring agents.

This food is alien to our systems and does not resemble anything close to organic whole food. Processed foods contain little fiber which, in turn, supports a growing multimillion-dollar industry for fiber supplements!

The new techno-refined foods quickly became the staples of the affluent diet. As long as we gleaned enough daily vitamins, everyone assumed overprocessed foods were causing no harm.

Why Overprocessed Food Is Unhealthy

- Processing strips away anticancer agents like glutathione that cannot be obtained from any other source in your diet.
- Toxic products are formed by high heat.
- Processed food forms unnatural amino acids (lysinoalanine) that are toxic and known to disrupt the manufacture of DNA.
- Heating can form antinutritional products that interfere with utilization, absorption, transport, and digestion of nutrients.
- Plant fiber is degraded and removed from many food products.
- Irradiation of food is a very controversial process. Studies show that split products (so-called *radiolytic* products) are toxic in animals.

- Minerals are lost. Food processing techniques also strip important mineral contents.
- Fat is added. Processed foods have high levels of trans-fatty acids and other oxidized fats that are linked to causing heart disease and cancer.
- Excess sugar is added to processed foods for taste.
- Non-nutritive sweeteners used in some processed foods are linked to increased brain cancer and hyperactivity in children.
- Processing of food is known to form substances that cause allergies.

This much seems clear: The American convenience food diet has played a role in the most common causes of premature death—cardio-vascular disease and cancer. And some pioneering studies have gradually convinced nutritionists to realize that there is much more to a good diet than adding vitamins and minerals to processed foods.

In the 1960s, as the term "health food" came into vogue, what was meant was that this food was more healthful than the processed, refined foods already on supermarket shelves. One of the early popular health foods was yogurt; the marketing campaign used spry elderly Soviet Georgians to extol its health benefits. Perceived as refreshing and exotic, yogurt was quickly accepted by consumers. In reality yogurt is just another dairy product.

In the mid 1970s, the fiber revolution hit the affluent diet. Scientific evidence suggested what many already knew—that non-nutritive or nondigestible fiber prevented colon cancer and was an important part of one's diet.

Now we have entered the era of chemopreventive foods—whole fresh foods—and seem to have gone full cycle. There are stunning indications that a number of chemopreventive plant chemicals are present naturally in our foods. Nature has provided us with a generous menu of phytochemicals (plant chemicals), which have demonstrated chemopreventive benefits.

Chemopreventive Agents
This is a good place to define terms:

- *Chemopreventive agent*—a non-nutritive substance that has demonstrated protection against cancer

- *Phytochemical*—a plant substance that has shown biological activity
- *Designer food*—a food that is processed or supplemented with chemopreventive substances
- *Functional food*—a unique food or food group that has potent chemopreventive properties

But how are phytochemicals likely to prevent cancer? The promotion of optimal health with non-nutritive substances sounds odd. But when you think about it, it's not surprising since the active ingredient for 25 percent of the planet's prescription drugs are substances originally extracted from plants. Not all plant chemicals are associated with chemoprevention, and for the purposes of this book we will only refer to the plant chemicals that have demonstrated chemoprevention.

These days we are tempted by health food, junk food, and health-junk foods like potato chips produced with no fat but loaded with salt. Some food companies are producing designer foods, processed or supplemented with chemopreventive agents such as vitamin C-enriched oranges or fiber-supplemented baked products. And now designer fats are hitting the market, fake fats that satisfy your craving for fat without adding inches to your waist and clogging your arteries.

Clearly you can survive without cancer-exterminating agents in your diet; they are not necessary to sustain life. Yet scientific evidence has become overwhelming indicating they will help you to stay healthy.

For example, a recent study failed to show reduction in breast cancer rates after using the celebrated vitamins A, C, and E. However the study did show significant protection from breast cancer with a continual infusion of vegetables. Other studies have shown that orange and tomato extracts that have been stripped of vitamin C still exhibit robust anticancer power.

It is becoming clear that dietary factors other than vitamins and minerals play an even more crucial role than traditionally acclaimed vitamins. Antioxidants 300 times more powerful than vitamin E have been found in beans, soy products, and seed oils. And recent experimental studies concur that switching from the traditional Japanese diet yields a subsequent rise of colon and prostate cancer—hallmarks of the affluent diet.

Another cancer combatant is chlorophyll, the green pigment found in dark green plants and a necessary component of photosynthesis. Chlorophyll and related compounds are recognized as being responsible for most of the antitoxic activity of certain vegetable extracts. For example, charbroiling food creates compounds that attack DNA, yet chlorophyll blocks the toxicity. If you consume foods rich in chlorophyll during a meal of charbroiled meat, it is claimed that the chlorophyll will not be absorbed and will remain present during the entire process of digestion, thereby blocking formation of toxic agents.

Fill your diet with cancer-crushing mixtures and your DNA will be less likely to get sliced, diced, and pulverized with above normal mutations.

Eat More Plants

Plants predate animals by millions of years, and they actually adapt better to environmental stress. Plants make all the antioxidant vitamins they need. But humans, who have either lost this ability or never had it, must rely on plants for their antioxidant vitamins. *So if you do nothing else, eat a plant-based diet.* The National Cancer Institute and other leading health agencies promote the simple act of eating more fruits and vegetables. This won't provide optimal protection. Ideally you should regularly consume an array of foods from the Super Eight Food Groups, since they contain a rich menu of cancer-busting agents. Nutritionists of the future will expand beyond the traditional food groups as we know them to recommend cancer-suppressing food groups as well.

It is important to eat foods that contain plant chemicals, not artificial dietary supplements. Unlike vitamins, phytochemicals should not be taken in the pill form found at the store. Eat whole organic foods rather than quick-cooking processed foods. Fresh food is better than frozen, and frozen food is better than canned.

We need to understand the role chemopreventives play in a healthy diet as well as we now understand the role of vitamins and minerals. The relatively few vitamins and minerals that exist each have precisely defined nutritional roles. In contrast tens of thousands of potentially important anticancer collages are present in whole foods.

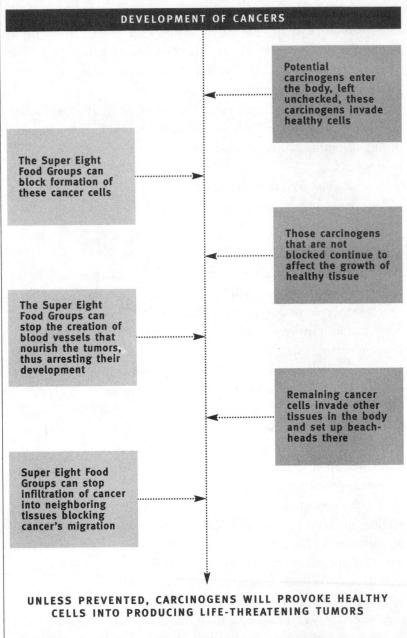

Figure 7

Chemopreventive food groups confer significant health benefits in ways that are not duplicated by other food groups. Each food group provides unique types of chemoprevention. The truth is, a cornucopia of fresh, whole foods and ingredients is available to the American consumer. Learn to eat wisely from the cancer-busting food groups to achieve maximum defense against the many diseases of the affluent diet.

SUPER EIGHT FOOD GROUPS	
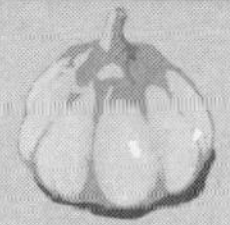	**1. Onion Group**—onion, garlic, asparagus
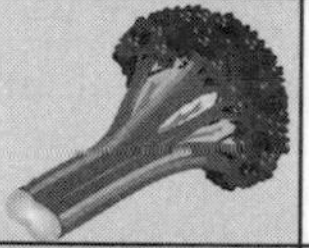	**2. Cruciferous Group**—broccoli, cabbage, cauliflower
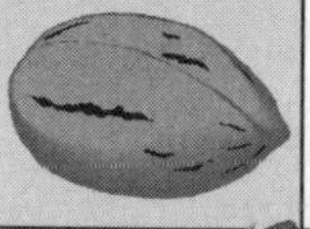	**3. Nuts & Seeds**—pumpkin seeds, sesame seeds, walnuts
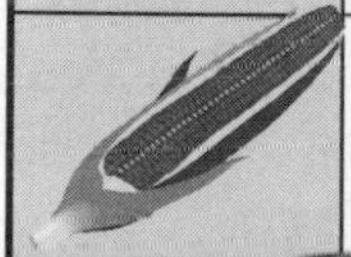	**4. Grass Group**—corn, oats, rice, wheat
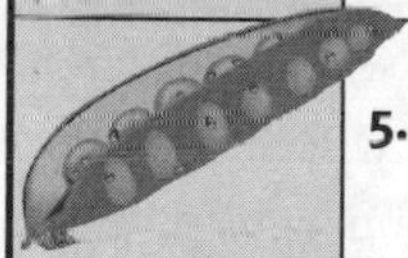	**5. Legume Group**—soybeans (tofu), green and wax beans, peas
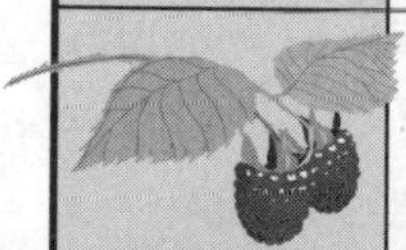	**6. Fruit**—citrus fruits, berries
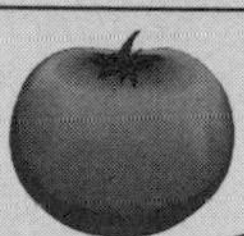	**7. Solanace Group**—tomatoes, potatoes
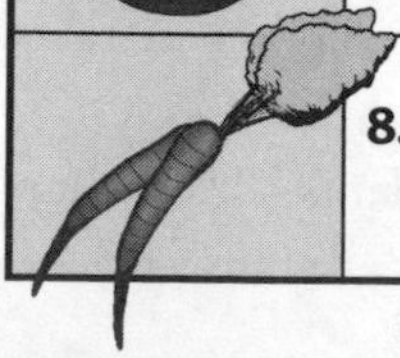	**8. Umbelliferous Group**—carrots, celery

Figure 4

Super Eight Food Groups

Onion Group

Since the beginning of civilization allium plants such as onion and garlic have been valued for their distinct flavors and medicinal properties. Inhabitants of the Middle and Far East have cultivated allium plants for at least 5,000 years. Ancient Egypt, China, and India all held onion and garlic in high regard; in Egypt pharaohs' burial chambers often contain dried relics of garlic cloves and wooden models of onions.

Recent human studies from China and Italy demonstrate that consumption of allium plants reduces stomach cancer. An area in the People's Republic of China, where cancer rates are high, shows a surprising reduction in stomach cancer when consumption of allium plants is high.

Garlic was recognized for its legendary medicinal uses long ago in the writings of Hippocrates and Aristotle. For many years it has also been known to decrease the growth of bacteria. In the 19th century French scientist Louis Pasteur investigated the antibacterial activities of garlic. More recently garlic has attracted the attention of modern scientists who are reconfirming many of its medicinal and cancer-stifling properties.

When crushed, garlic cloves liberate over seventy different sulfur compounds, which is where it gets its pungent scent (garlic is sometimes referred to as the stinking rose). A good percentage of garlic's protective qualities hinge on the many sulfur-containing compounds that are not liberated until the cloves are crushed. Once crushed many of these compounds enter the air as gases, and once airborne they are gone, which is one reason many of the cancer-demolishing materials have not been successfully isolated. Some of these may never be isolated since they are so unstable once they've been removed from the plant. Therefore, if you ingest pills and extracts you will not receive the full safeguarding benefits of garlic.

Nature has provided an abundance of onion plants—more than 600 species—including the common plants garlic, onions, chives, leeks, shallots, and scallions.

Onions provide the richest source of *quercetin,* a potent and versatile anticancer, disease-hindering flavonoid. Yellow and red onions are a good source of quercetin, though white onions are not. More than 135 slightly different quercetin compounds exist, such as rutin, which is used to treat fragile capillaries (tiny blood vessels). Quercetin is the most abundant flavonol in red wine, where rutin is also present. As a rule the deeply red Cabernet Sauvignon has the highest quercetin content. Other dietary sources include broccoli, red grapes, shallots, and yellow squash.

Anticancer Benefits of the Onion Group
A number of qualities recommend the foods in this group. All of them:
- Are antimicrobial
- Prevent tumors
- Lower risk of stroke (decrease platelet sticking)
- Lower nitrosamine formation
- Lower lipids
- Inhibit cancers (skin, stomach, liver, colon, lung, cervix)
- Block formation of cancer-causing compounds (nitrosamine)
- Inhibit chemical toxicity such as acetaminophen and tobacco
- Inhibit prostaglandins that play a role in cancer

HEALTH BENEFITS OF QUERCETIN

anticancer
antioxidant
anti-inflammatory
antibacterial
antiviral
antifungal
lessens allergies and asthma
may protect from heart disease

Cruciferous Group
For thousands of years cruciferous vegetables have been used for food, and used medicinally to treat gout, diarrhea, stomach ailments, headaches, mushroom poisoning, and to promote wound healing. The crucifer flowers are cross-shaped (*crucis* is Latin for cross). Cruciferous vegetables refer to foods of the cabbage family and commonly include broccoli, brussels sprouts, cabbage, cauliflower, garden cress, radish, turnips, and watercress.

The cruciferous vegetables contain many cancer-slashing compounds, including the major class of compounds called *glucosino-*

lates. Glucosinolates are a class of more than 100 sulfur-containing compounds, the vast majority of which show anticancer activity.

A number of protective glucosinolates are released from cruciferous vegetables when the plant is chopped or chewed (fresh crucifers are preferred). Watercress, a popular item in Asian diets, is very high in *phenethyl isothiocyanate* (PEITC) and *indole-3-carbinol* (I3C); compounds, which have been shown to inhibit lung tumors. Even more encouraging are human studies showing that lower cancer rates generally correlate with frequent consumption of cruciferous vegetables. A constant infusion of garlic and cruciferous vegetables is specifically associated with reduced colon cancer.

ANTICANCER BENEFITS OF CRUCIFEROUS VEGETABLES

protect DNA

increase detoxification

may prevent cancers of the breast, prostate, lung, throat, stomach, and colon

block chemical toxicity (aflatoxin)

Nut and Seed Group

Seeds and nuts are especially cancer-bashing because they contain strong antioxidants in order to maintain the viability of the seed. A seed is part of a flowering plant that contains an embryo. Nuts such as hazelnuts and chestnuts are actually a single-seeded dry fruit. Brazil nuts are not true nuts either but are seeds, as are almonds, pecans, walnuts, and coconuts. Legumes are in the seed family and include peanuts, beans, and peas.

Some of the antioxidants in these seed foods have not been chemically characterized, while others, such as those found in the azuki bean, are more potent than vitamin E. Antioxidants in the lotus seed preserve its ability to germinate for over 2,000 years!

Today many of the cancer-pulverizing properties of nuts and seeds are thought to be the result of protease inhibitors. A *protease* is an enzyme, a fancy name for a specialized protein that accelerates specific chemical reactions. Life as we know it would not exist without enzymes. A protease specifically works on proteins by breaking them down. Tumor cells need proteases in order to migrate and invade distant sites, increasing blood vessel production and cell division. Currently protease inhibitors are being used as a treatment for AIDS.

Compounds that block the action of proteases, or *protease inhibitors*, are packed into virtually all seeds. Rice, corn, and beans contain protease inhibitors, and their consumption can lower incidences of breast, colon, and prostate cancer. Since seeds contain high concentrations of protease inhibitors, they may limit the occurrence of these cancers in humans. Continuing experiments have shown that protease inhibitors also hinder tumor development and can reduce the size of tumors as well.

FOODS HIGH IN
PROTEASE INHIBITORS

fruits—bananas

nuts—oil and seeds

legumes—chick peas and soybeans

cereals—barley, rye, oats

cucumber seeds

squash

zucchini

corn

potatoes

rice

Sesame seeds are one of the oldest oilseeds known to humans. The sesame seed and its oil have long been extolled for their nutritious medicinal effects, including their ability to increase energy and prevent aging. Traditionally sesame oil has been recognized as being very stable against turning rancid. Sesame oil antioxidants have shown antiaging effects, and sesame oil components work together with vitamin E to suppress disease.

When heated, sesame seed oil produces large amounts of sesamol, a more potent antioxidant compound than that found in native sesame seed oil. Fried foods in the traditional Japanese diet hamper cancer, as compared to the Western diet, because the Japanese use sesame seed oil, which the frying process converts into potent antioxidant compounds. Remember, the many toxic components formed during cooking provide some of the risks of indulging in Western-style food.

Grasses Group

Grains such as oats and wheat have marked inhibitory effects in the presence of carcinogens. That protection is due to fiber and to components associated with fiber, such as lignans.

If you recall, *lignans* are a major structural constituent of plants. Having a wide range of biological activities, they are antitumor and antiviral. Lignan-rich plants have an interesting history as active ingredients in many diverse cultures, including Chinese medicine.

The structural similarity between lignans and estrogens has led many to speculate on the role lignans may serve in humans. In humans, lignans bind weakly to estrogen receptors. Studies have shown that women who have breast cancer excrete lower amounts of lignans than healthy women do. Many researchers have made the obvious speculation: Low incidences of breast cancer may be due to the presence of lignans from a fiber-rich diet. It could be that lignans have an antiestrogen effect and suppress the growth of cancer.

The primary sources for lignans are flax seed (linseed), rye, buckwheat, soy, millet, oats, and barley.

Legume Group

One serving of soy each day can keep cancer away! Because soybeans are excellent sources of protein, they have been consumed for thousands of years. In East Asia soy forms a significant part of the diet, starting from early childhood. And in Asia, incidence of breast cancer and colon cancer is considerably lower than in the West. Vegetarians who consume soybean-based products in place of meat also have lower rates of breast and colon cancer.

An exciting study recently showed a 50 percent reduction in breast cancer among women who consumed only a fraction of an ounce (55 milligrams) of soy protein every day. While these studies do not conclusively prove soybeans are causing this lowered rate, the results are consistent with the trend showing that soybean intake reduces cancer risk. It's helpful to note that soy flour and soy concentrates are rich sources of soy; however, soy sauce and soy oils are not.

Soybeans are proving to be antiviral, anticancer, antifungal, and antioxidant protease inhibitors. And soy seems to reduce cholesterol levels as well.

Among the edible legumes, soybeans contain the highest amounts of *saponins*. Soya saponins are a diverse family of cancer-zapping chemicals, which are structurally similar to the primary chemopreventive ingredient in licorice. Saponins, which are toxic to tumor cells, inhibit DNA synthesis in tumor cells, thereby decreasing tumor cell growth.

People in Asian countries consume many fermented soybean products. Fermented soy products, such as soy sauce, are also anti-nutritious to cancer, and since they provide excellent sources of digestible protein they are often used as meat substitutes in Japanese diets. Fermentation, with its numerous chemical reactions, forms many new substances, including flavors and aromas.

Fermented soybean products such as miso, natto, and tempeh are high in vitamin B12 and have potent antioxidant activity. *Miso*, a popular seasoning, which is created by fermenting soybeans and rice, is one of Asia's most important foods. When the Chinese first discovered this remarkable delicacy they reserved it exclusively for the nobility. Miso later became a staple food of the Orient, used for over 2,000 years. *Natto* is a typical soybean food in Japan, made by fermenting steamed soybeans and the bacteria *Bacillus natto*. Traditional natto is eaten with hot rice, soy sauce, and mustard. *Tempeh* is another fermented soy product (made from the fungus *Rhizopus oligosporous*) and is quite popular in Indonesia.

Fruit Group

In the distant past humans practiced such a long tradition of eating vitamin C-rich foods (such as fruit) that eventually our bodies lost the ability to manufacture vitamin C. Many citrus fruits contain a wide variety of cancer-curbing compounds, including citrus oils, glutathione, folic acid, and certainly vitamin C. The biological activity of citrus juice flavonoids covers a broad spectrum, including anticarcinogenic and antitumor activities. You will recall that flavonoids prevent the invasion of cancer cells, and they also potently inhibit tumor cell growth. Literature reporting the vitamin-like activities of flavonoids has recently dramatically increased.

ANTICANCER BENEFITS OF FLAVONOIDS

anti-inflammatory

antiallergy

anticancer

antiviral

anti-tumor

antioxidant

prevent tumor cell invasion

A variety of cancer-arresting fruit oils, called *monoterpenes*, are found in grapefruit, lemon, lime, sweet orange, bitter orange, and bergamot oils. Grapefruit juice contains a flavonoid compound called *naringin*. Naringin has been demonstrated to protect from a mold toxin (aflatoxin) that causes liver toxicity. A common citrus oil, limonene (the major component of lemon and orange peel oil), is also present in caraway, thyme, cardamom, and orange flower. Citrus liminoids are known to induce anticancer activities.

Eight different liminoids have been found to increase the activity of the enzyme *glutathione-S-transferase (GST)*. GST is a detoxifying enzyme from the liver that speeds reactions with highly reactive chemicals called electrophiles, thus forming less toxic varieties that are then removed in the urine. Because most carcinogens operate via a reactive intermediate, increasing GST is believed to be a major means of deactivating carcinogens. Liver enzymes are continually converting some chemicals into a chain of tiny disasters. Meanwhile, the enzyme GST is turning carcinogens into harmless chemicals.

AGENTS THAT INCREASE DETOXIFYING ACTIVITY (GST)

citrus fruits

broccoli, garlic, cauliflower, cabbage

celery seed oil

magnesium

low-protein and high-carbohydrate diet

Over the last few years the vital importance of GST has become widely recognized. GSTs detoxify a diverse array of potentially carcinogenic chemicals, thereby preventing a reaction with essential constituents of the cell (namely the DNA). Therefore, compounds that increase GST will probably protect from cancer.

To keep GST humming along, you need a cofactor called glutathione. Fresh, uncooked foods contain the most glutathione; canned and processed foods are largely stripped of it. Cooking can also dramatically reduce glutathione levels. Glutathione rich foods include: watermelon, asparagus, avocado, strawberries, peaches, broccoli, tomatoes, squash, okra, white potatoes, cauliflower, grapefruit, and oranges.

In turn, glutathione production is influenced by two magnesium-dependent enzymes, and it requires cysteine as well. Magnesium-rich foods include: spinach, watermelon, peanuts, bananas, cantaloupe, honeydew melon, and beans.

Since glutathione is a required cofactor, any depletion can risk serious toxicity. One example is acetaminophen, a common painkiller that may cause dramatic reductions in levels of glutathione.

Raspberries, strawberries, and blackberries may be better for your health than was formerly realized. Besides being vitamin-rich, berries may inhibit cancer with *tannins* (the bitter agents found in tea, fruits, and the bark of trees).

Ellagic acid is a tannin found naturally in many fruits and berries, and it is chemopreventive for lung cancer. Many fruits contain ellagic acid, including pomegranate, blackberries, strawberries, and raspberries. It is thought that ellagic acid binds to cancer-producing chemicals, thus rendering them inactive. The amount of tannin found in berries is five to six times higher than that found in plums, pears, and apples.

Solanace Group

A tomato a day will keep cancer away! The solanace group includes tomatoes, potatoes, sweet potatoes, and beets. An interesting study recently showed a reduced rate of prostate cancer in men who frequently consumed baked tomato products in pasta dishes. New studies with tomato juice extracts identify several substances that can inhibit the formation of carcinogens. In fact, even after the vitamin C was totally removed, tomato extracts still showed potent inhibiting properties. The whole tomato was much more effective against the formation of cancer than the vitamin C component alone—yet another example suggesting that whole foods are powerful arsenals in the war against cancer.

Umbelliferous Group

Naturally bioactive products occur widely in umbelliferous plants, which include: carrots, celery, parsley, dill, celeriac, parsnips, lovage, angelica root, anise, cumin, chervil, fennel, caraway, and coriander. Umbelliferous vegetables are extremely rich sources of plant chemicals. Phytochemicals are present in relatively high amounts in celery seed oil, and in fresh celery as well (in fact these are responsible for conferring the characteristic odor of celery).

Celery compounds also modify the detoxifying enzyme GST. For example, celery seed oil contains five natural products, many of which increase the activity of GST fivefold. Even more convincing data in studies with mice showed that celery seed oil decreased the number of mice with tumors, as well as the number of tumors per mouse.

Numerous animal and human studies indicate that carrots (carotenoids) inhibit cancer and have anticarcinogenic properties. The vast majority of studies have focused on beta carotene, though more recently attention has been given to other compounds, such as lycopene and canthaxanthin. It has been shown that over forty different carotenoids are commonly found in fruits and vegetables.

There also is growing evidence suggesting that high intakes of green and yellow vegetables offer protection from cancer. The cancers protected against by members of the *Umbelliferae* family include: mouth, gastric tract, colon, lung, lining of uterus, pancreas, prostate, and bladder.

It should be noted that plants are composed of thousands of different chemicals, and food is a complex mixture. So the results of experimental studies with animals may not always agree with human studies.

Other Cancer-Crushing Agents

Spices

Licorice has been used as a crude drug since ancient times. The sweet root of the flowering pea, or licorice, has been used as an antidote to poisons, as a means of soothing irritations, as an elixir, and as medicine in China for thousands of years. Egyptians believed licorice would give the newly dead powers to ward off evil spirits.

Traditionally licorice has been used not only as a medicine but also as a food additive, due to its sweetness and flavoring properties. Licorice is a root extract widely used by the food industry as a sweetening agent in candy, chewing gum, chocolate, liquors, and beer.

HEALTH BENEFITS OF LICORICE

antimicrobial

antioxidant

antitumor

anti-inflammatory

antiulcer

anticancer

increases detox (GST)

The main licorice constituent is used to treat stomach ulcers. Licorice is anticancer and protects from chemical toxicity. But the fundamental effect associated with decreased cancer is its inhibition of the enzyme ODC (ornithine decarboxylase), which may be very useful in preventing skin, bladder, breast, and prostate cancer.

ODC inhibitors include: licorice, carrots, wheat, garlic, onions, asparagus, cucumbers, tomatoes, radishes, potatoes, strawberries, citrus, cruciferous vegetables, and spices like turmeric.

Rosemary and sage are remarkably potent antioxidants. In fact, many herbs and spices are naturally rich in antioxidants.

Cayenne pepper (capsicum) is an extremely hot spice—so hot that a concentrated version of it is used in the weapon pepper spray. At lower doses cayenne protects against stomach ulcers, decreases platelet aggregation, and hinders the formation of strokes (antithrombotic).

Curcumin is a plant spice and a major yellow coloring agent. The dried, powdered form is known as turmeric, used as one of the major coloring agents in curry. Turmeric has been used for centuries as a spice, food colorant, and food preservative. Turmeric can block cancer, acting as an antioxidant or anti-inflammatory agent.

Precaution: Avoid turmeric compounds in your diet if you have allergies or autoimmune diseases since consumption of curcumin may aggravate the symptoms.

Ginger root, with its sweet aroma and pungent taste, is widely used as a spice. It is also known to contain some very potent antioxidant compounds. Most of the isolated compounds from ginger exhibit even stronger antioxidant properties than vitamin E. Ginger is a potent antioxidant that can inhibit blood clots (platelet clumping).

ANTIOXIDANT SPICES

allspice, basil, bay leaf

caradamom, cinnamon, cloves, cumin

fennel, ginger

mace, marjoram, nutmeg

oregano, perilla, rosemary, sage

thyme, turmeric

Tea

Since ancient times tea has been associated with maintaining body and soul. About 800 years ago the Japanese Buddhist priest Eisai wrote a book called *Tea Drinking for Health.* In its first paragraph he described tea as a *wonder drug for health.*

Though tea has been cultivated in the Far East for thousands of years, only recently have scientists isolated tea polyphenols and tea extracts. These have now been shown to prevent food from turning rancid, to prevent infections in the intestinal tract, and to contribute to a decreased rate of respiratory and cardiovascular diseases and cancer.

The major tea phytochemicals are *catechin* from green tea and *thea flavins* from black tea. Tea extracts also protect against radiation, and they lower cholesterol and blood pressure levels as well.

For a long time tea has been considered effective in mitigating diarrhea caused by bacterial infections. Human studies show lower risks of gastric cancer among those who drink large quantities of green tea.

In Japan many products such as candy, toothpaste, and beverages have been enriched with green tea extracts (Sunphenon). Green tea has also been discovered to inhibit cavity-producing bacteria.

Tea polyphenols (broadly tannins) are known to have a strong affinity to proteins. When we drink tea this is felt on our palates as astringency, or what some refer to as cotton mouth.

Drink Away Cancer With Tea!

Green and black teas are derived from the leaf of the bush *Camellia sinensis*. After tea is picked, the leaves are left to wither and dry in the hot air. Black tea is put through a process of oxidation, which imparts its dark color and flavorful aroma.

In making green tea the fresh leaves are steamed, which destroys the enzymes that cause fermentation in black tea. Since green tea is not allowed to oxidize like black tea, green tea has a fresh grassy quality, as well as unique polyphenols that are able to be preserved in the final product.

DISEASE PREVENTION BENEFITS OF TEA		
	GREEN TEA	BLACK TEA
blocks mutagens	●[1]	
antioxidant	●[3]	●[2]
antibacterial	●[4]	●
anticancer	●[5]	
antivirus	●[6]	●[6]
antipromoter	●	
antiaging properties	●	
reduces allergies	●	
protects against radiation	●	
lowers blood pressure	●	●
blocks nitrosamine formation	●	●

[1] Oolong tea suppresses chromosome damage.
[2] Greater than vitamin E.
[3] Twenty times more potent than vitamin E.
[4] Inhibits dental caries.
[5] Colon, throat, skin, and prostate cancer. Green tea protects from many chemically-caused cancers.
[6] Influenza virus.

Potassium

Hardly anyone notices the cancer-hindering effects of potassium, and a scarcity of reports on it reflect this. However a number of human and other animal studies have suggested that potassium can eradicate cancer.

Potassium is the most common, positively charged ion inside a cell. In contrast, sodium is the main, positively charged ion on the outside of a cell. Very simply put, potassium is an insider, and as such it plays a vital role in grooming the DNA and keeping it happy.

For a million years humans have eaten high potassium/ low sodium diets. Our bodies were designed for this from the very start, based on our hunting and gathering diet. Only recently, through our highly processed foods, have we begun receiving far more sodium than potassium in our diets.

In general, high dietary potassium, as well as high blood levels of potassium, have been associated with less cancer and decreased growth of tumors. Recent revelations in Seneca County, New York, showed that people there had unexpectedly low rates of most cancers. These low rates are thought to result from the unique geological formations of the region, characterized by higher amounts of potassium salts in the water and the soil. Animal studies show that when water is supplemented with potassium chloride, this decreases the incidence of digestive tract tumors. The reverse is also true: a higher sodium-to-potassium ratio is associated with greater incidence of cancer.

> *The wisdom of nature, honed by thousands of years of physiological adaptations to a naturally high potassium intake, should not be lightly dismissed.*
>
> —Kaplan, N. M., and C. V. S. Ram. Potassium supplements for hypertension. *N Engl J Med* 1990; 322:623–624.

Several other factors may be at play in relation to salt and increased gastric cancers. Table salt (sodium chloride) is known to irritate the stomach lining and to promote digestive tract tumors in rats.

Exactly how potassium hinders cancer is unclear. What we do know is that altered surface properties of tumor cells may result in uncontrolled growth, and that potassium plays an important role with DNA, including assisting in cell communication. It is theorized that cells that lack potassium may be responsible for distorted genetic information in the DNA. On the other hand, high potassium levels can transform the DNA's shape back to normal.

Studies show that decreased cancer rates are linked to increased consumption of high-potassium foods including: avocados, bananas, oranges, cantaloupe, honeydew melons, tomato juice, spinach, potatoes, watermelon, and pumpkin.

Aspirin

Aspirin, which is contained in willow tree bark, has been used for centuries as a remedy for pain, fever, and inflammation. Only recently, partly because of its effects on the blood, has aspirin been found to prevent heart attacks, strokes, and certain cancers. It is now believed that women can help prevent breast cancer by taking aspirin every three days. Human studies show that aspirin decreases both colon and rectal cancers. In fact the American Cancer Society reports that colon cancer death rates are 50 percent lower in people who use aspirin regularly.

Aspirin may play an extremely important role in cancer by blocking production of prostaglandins, inhibiting tumor growth, and enhancing the immune response.

Many fruits and vegetables naturally contain aspirin (salicylates): apples, apricots, cherries, grapes, peaches, plums, berries, cucumbers, peppers, and tomatoes.

Precaution: People with aspirin-induced asthma should try to avoid these foods. Also, if you plan to use aspirin regularly, make sure to take it with a meal and use an enteric-coated variety to prevent irritation of the digestive tract.

Fruits From the Sea

The Japanese use a variety of dried seaweed and marine algae in their dishes. Several edible species such as the lobe leaf, seaweed, and sea tangles have significant antitumor and antioxidant activities.

Marine algae are well known to be stable against oxidation after they have been dried and stored, despite the fact that they have a high content of unsaturated fatty acids. For example, green algae and brown algae show potent antioxidant activity, supporting the importance of eating whole foods.

Methyl Groups

A methyl group is a simple chemical mixture made up of one carbon atom and three hydrogen atoms. Methyl groups are needed for the repair and assembly of DNA and other vital cell components. Dietary supply from the methyl groups plays a crucial role in preventing cancer.

Dietary sources of methyl groups come from the amino acids methionine and choline and are found in foods such as: soy products, rice, peanuts, pecans, oatmeal, fish, meats, and egg yolks.

Proper methyl function requires the additional nutrients folic acid and vitamin B12.

Folic Acid-rich Foods

- Dark green leafy vegetables, especially collard greens, spinach, romaine lettuce
- Brussels sprouts, and beets
- Lentils and soybeans
- Many other fresh fruits and vegetables, especially oranges, grapefruit, asparagus, peas, avocados, and broccoli
- Navy beans
- Nuts
- Whole wheat products

Processed foods that are cooked or canned will destroy folic acid.

SUBSTANCES VITAL TO DNA REPAIR

vitamins, B3, B6, B12

folic acid

choline, methionine

low-fat diets (less damage to DNA)

magnesium, zinc, potassium

Mineral Supplements

Recently there has been enormous publicity surrounding trace metals and essential minerals.

Organically grown produce has been shown to contain up to three times more minerals and trace elements than commercial produce. As noted earlier, maintaining a proper mineral balance can avoid the uptake of toxic agents like cadmium, lead, and mercury.

If you suspect either an excess or a deficiency in essential or trace metals, or if you are concerned about heavy metal exposure, a metal analysis of your hair may be the first place to start. A company specializing in trace metal analysis of hair samples is listed in appendix F. Should you take colloidal minerals? See appendix B.

Essential minerals or trace elements play critical roles in health and nutrition. Life evolved in a soup of inorganic elements. Life has used minerals as signals, and also as catalysts that speed up the reactions of life (that is, metabolism). By maintaining a proper mineral balance you can avoid the uptake of some toxic agents. Determining which minerals are necessary for proper health was first studied in the early 1900s, but unraveling the biochemical roles these minerals play did not occur until recently. The number of trace minerals recognized to be essential has rapidly increased since the late 1940s. Over the last thirty years minerals have been shown to play key roles in almost every step of life's functions.

Mineral deficiencies can occur from consuming an overprocessed diet.

Food Sources of Minerals

- Boron (garlic and onions)
- Calcium (dark leafy vegetables, widely distributed in dairy products—not a recommended source)
- Chromium (spices such as black pepper, broccoli, prunes, raisins, peanuts and nuts, asparagus, brewer's yeast, beer, wine, wheat, wheat germ)
- Cobalt (oysters, clams, poultry, and milk)[2]
- Copper (shellfish, asparagus, nuts, whole grain cere raisins, apples, broccoli)
- Fluorine (spinach, peas, beets, whole wheat bread, sweet potatoes)
- Germanium (garlic and onions)
- Iodine (seafood, seaweed, iodized salt)
- Iron (red meat—not a recommended source—black strap molasses, potatoes, kidney beans, tofu, dark green vegetables, cereals)
- Lithium (tomatoes, mushrooms, cucumbers, red cabbage, black tea, paprika, marjoram)
- Magnesium (nuts, legumes, cereal grains, chocolate, green vegetables, potatoes)
- Manganese (avocados, unrefined cereals, dark bread, tea, ginger, nuts, seeds, beets, turnip greens, green leafy vegetables)
- Molybdenum (legumes, cereal, yeast)
- Nickel (oats and cabbage)

MINERALS

essential minerals—sodium, potassium, calcium, magnesium, phosphorus, chloride

trace elements—cobalt, chromium, copper, iron, iodine, manganese, molybdenum, selenium

controversial trace elements—arsenic, lead,[1] lithium, nickel, silicon, vanadium, fluorine, tin

---

[1] No one should supplement with lead. Because of widespread pollution the challenge lies in preventing exposure.

[2] Never take cobalt as a supplement (such as cobalt sulfate) because it causes toxicity to the heart (cardiomyopathy). When cobalt was used as a foam stabilizer in the 1960s, heavy beer drinkers suffered irreversible damage to their heart muscles.

- Phosphorus (seeds, nuts, legumes, grains)
- Potassium (vegetables, cabbage, spinach, molasses, peas, bananas, fruit, bran flakes, cocoa)
- Selenium (cereals, garlic, nuts, seafood, wheat, bran, soybeans)
- Silicon (unrefined grains, oats, wheat bran, soybeans, beets, leafy vegetables, brown rice)
- Tin (fruits, vegetables, juices)
- Vanadium (fish, green beans, whole grains, radishes)
- Zinc (whole grain products, oysters, nuts, seeds, green leafy vegetables)

Importance of Chemopreventive Agents

The toxic substances in our environment, whether they occur naturally or are human-made, can cause considerable strain on our natural defenses and on our elimination pathways. It has been estimated that each cell of our body is pelted with over 100,000 oxidative hits per day. Every day a typical human cell sustains 5,000 mutations. In theory any one of these mutations could lead to cancer. This usually does not occur since most mutations do not take place in both strands of genetic material that make up DNA. Remember, DNA is structurally similar to a train track. If both tracks are damaged in the same area, then DNA is hard to repair.

Some DNA inevitably sustain damage; we have few natural defenses to protect ourselves from the myriad toxic substances in our environment. One example of a natural defense is the constant shedding of skin and of the cells lining our gastrointestinal system. Some intestinal tract cells are shed at such high rates that it makes little difference if they have mutated.

A number of systems will protect against the toxic effects of carcinogens. Remember, DNA-altering chemicals and radioactivity change genetic material, which may then lead to cancer. But your cells can repair DNA by scanning the entire length of the strands, then removing and correcting mistakes in the DNA.

In order to maintain optimal and lasting health, to keep our bodies precisely tuned and firing on all cylinders, dietary chemopreventive agents are absolutely necessary for everyone to include in their daily diet.

Chapter Recap

- Processed foods are alien to our systems. After having been processed, these foods do not contain the cancer protection found in traditional foods.

- Many cancer-suppressing agents are neither vitamins nor minerals; in fact they are not even nutrients. Yet you need them to stay healthy.

- We need to eat fresh whole foods that contain plant chemicals.

- When chemopreventive food groups are incorporated in a healthy diet, they not only confer significant health benefits, but they do so in a way that is unique and not duplicated by other food groups.

- Breast cancer is the leading cause of death for women between the ages 40 and 55. Each year in the United States more women die from breast cancer than all the American soldiers killed in the Vietnam war.

Cancer-Busting Regimen

The simple beauty behind the cancer-busting regimen is that everyone from every walk of life can receive its health benefits. From the moment you start the cancer-busting daily diet, you will be significantly enhancing your long-term health. Even better, it takes no additional effort to achieve the regimen's advantages, once you apply your new awareness in understanding cancer.

A man is rich in proportion to what he can do without.

—Henry David Thoreau, 1817–62

Strategies

What are the grand strategies behind the cancer-busting regimen? First, as discussed in the previous chapter, we must identify the naturally occurring agents found in foods from around the world that provide optimal cancer and illness suppression. Second, we must discover new methods of food preparation that minimize the creation of cancer-producing substances.

Each of the eight anticancer food groups provides a unique type of protection not often duplicated by other foods. Merely eating more fruits and vegetables is not likely to provide optimal protection. Rather, a collection of cancer-busting foods from the Super Eight Food Groups must be introduced into your diet daily.

The Super Eight Food Groups

1. Onion group—garlic, onions, asparagus
2. Cruciferous group—broccoli, cabbage, cauliflower
3. Nuts and seeds group—pumpkin seeds, sesame seeds, walnuts
4. Grass group—corn, oats, rice, wheat
5. Legume group—soybeans, green and wax beans, peas
6. Fruit group—citrus fruits, berries
7. Solanace group—tomatoes and potatoes
8. Umbelliferous group—carrots and celery

Tips for Success

- Every day include fresh choices from as many of the Super Eight Food Groups as possible. Do not accept canned and processed foods that have been stripped of chemopreventive agents, nor the false assurances of pills and extracts.
- Ideally, stick to the cancer-busting regimen all the time. But if you cannot, only deviate on the weekends.
- Try to consume a plant-based diet rather than a meat-based diet.
- Do not eat overcooked or burnt foods or foods cooked at searing temperatures. Preferred cooking methods include steaming, broiling, microwaving, and light baking.
- For cooking use only sesame seed, olive, or macadamia nut oil.
- Take daily vitamin supplements, especially beta carotene, vitamins B12, time-release C, E, and selenium.

Cancer-Free Food Preparation

The way food is prepared can have a major impact on the amount of cancer-producing chemicals formed in that food. Recommended methods of food preparation: steaming, poaching, light oven broiling, low-temperature roasting or baking, microwaving, or light boiling.

Avoid overcooking meat, chicken, fish, or any food. Especially avoid charbroiled and fried foods. When you grill or charbroil you introduce a number of undesirable substances into your foods. The sooty black char that forms on food from charbroiling or frying is a complex mixture of chemicals, including burnt proteins and carcinogenic compounds, and these compounds have been linked to both heart disease and cancer. When you do grill, use a soy flour-based marinade.

Fried foods are subjected to high temperatures, and they contain considerably more compounds that are damaging to DNA than non-fried foods. Studies have shown that people who consume too many fried foods such as bacon show pulverized products of their DNA in their urine.

If you can't live without fried or charbroiled foods, make sure you remove the black char from cooked food, and block the meat from direct exposure to flames and smoke by using aluminum foil or other baking materials. Avoid eating the outer layer or the skin of poultry.

Ways to Reduce Toxic Agents in Cooked Food

When you cook meat, several methods will reduce toxic agents. If you must fry or charbroil, first partially cook the meat in a microwave oven, then discard the resulting liquid that forms from the meat. Three minutes in a microwave oven before frying can block up to 94 percent of the toxic mutagens. However, the clear liquid that results from microwave heating is suspected to contain compounds that are converted into damaging mutagens. There are other ways of reducing the formation of toxic substances from cooking:

- Coat food with soy flour or cottonseed flour before cooking.
- Cook at low temperatures.
- Reduce heating time to form less toxic agents.
- Use microwave precooking. Before frying or charbroiling, briefly microwave and discard the cooking juices.
- Block foods from direct contact with flames and charcoal.
- Reduce intake of outer *black char*. It is a source of the most powerful mutagens.
- Dietary fiber reduces the danger of eating cooked food as well. Fiber from corn and wheat bran lower the toxicity of charbroiled food when eaten together.

Here are other health protective foods to eat with charbroiled foods:

- Cruciferous vegetables counteract barbecued foods.
- Omega-3 fats also decrease toxicity of cooking mutagens.
- Chlorophyll, the plant pigment in green leafy vegetables, will reduce the toxicity of cooking mutagens.
- Tea extracts, especially green tea, may decrease toxicity.
- Burdock, a popular plant used in oriental cooking, may be beneficial.
- Antioxidant vitamins such as A, C, E, and beta carotene hinder cancer growth.

Cooking Oils

On your next visit to the grocery store, purchase a large bottle of sesame seed oil. Your DNA will thank you! For cooking purposes, olive oil burns at a lower temperature and is probably not as cancer-smashing as sesame oil, but it is still superior to corn, safflower, sunflower, or cottonseed oils. Macadamia nut oil is harder to obtain, but it is another good alternative. Canola oil contains essential fatty acids (EFAs), as does heart-protective fish oil.

Essential Fats

By eating carbohydrates the human body can make all of the different fats that it requires except for two: linoleic acid (omega-6), and linolenic acid (omega-3). A healthful diet requires both essential fats. However, if you eat a typical American diet you won't get enough of the omega-3 linolenic acid. And as you can see from the chart below the average person who uses corn, safflower, cotton seed, sunflower, and peanut oils gets an excess of omega-6 linoleic acid.

Since they must be supplied through the diet, these fats are termed essential. The essential fats (or fatty acids) are widely distributed in plant and seed oils. There is much debate concerning the best dietary ratio of linoleic acid to linolenic acid. At present the World Health Organization is recommending a ratio from 5:1 to 10:1.

ESSENTIAL FATTY ACIDS		
	LINOLEIC ACID (OMEGA-6)	LINOLENIC ACID (OMEGA-3)
flax seed (linseed)	●	●
walnuts and walnut oil	●	●
soybean oil and products	●	●
canola oil (grapeseed oil)	●	●
wheat germ oil		●
cottonseed and peanut oil	●	
sunflower seed oil	●	
corn and safflower oil	●	

There are more common dietary sources of linoleic than linolenic acid, so it is to be expected that most people are consuming too much linoleic acid. The first four sources of essential fatty acids (EFA) listed below—flax seed, walnut, soybean, and canola oils—contain both. Fish oils are high in the omega-3 fats called eicosapentaenoic acid (or EPA) and docosahexaenoic acid (or DHA). Fish that are especially high in EPA and DHA include: salmon, herring, mackerel, sablefish, sardines and tuna. Olive oil is an example of an omega-9 fat.

Delve into your pantry and discard all your omega-6 vegetable oils like corn, safflower, and cottonseed oils. Halt your consumption of, and generally avoid, partially hydrogenated vegetable oils. The process of hydrogenation is accomplished by bubbling hydrogen gas through oil, which produces trans-fatty acids. Recent human studies indicate that consumption of trans-fatty acids in margarine and shortenings may contribute to higher rates of cancer and heart disease. Food makers add these to improve the creaminess of a product, and to extend its shelf life. Some foods like pie crusts are packed with partially hydrogenated vegetable oils to achieve their flaky texture and taste. Be wary since food labels do not include the amount of trans-fatty acids. Food manufacturers need only list a total, along with the saturated fat content of the food.

Cut down on fried foods because oils and fats tend to oxidize at high temperatures (for example, in oil used for cooking french fries). Once ingested oxidized fats are guilty of a peculiar foam cell formation in blood vessels. Foam cells pave the way for cancer and heart disease.

Precautions

We're often careless or ignorant about the condition of the food we purchase and the ways we prepare it. Here are a few points to consider:

Moldy Foods

Any foods that have developed mold or fungal growth should not be eaten. Do not merely wash or cut the mold off, since potent fungal toxins will still be present in the food. Many foods by nature contain various molds, such as cheeses.

Other precautions:

- Wash food immediately before preparation.
- Store foods in watertight and airtight vacuum containers (not warm, moist conditions that encourage mold growth).
- Refrigerate foods to slow bacterial and fungal growth.
- Use foods two to three days from the date of purchase.
- Freeze leftover foods that will not be used immediately.

Food Additives

The Food and Drug Administration (FDA) has mandated toxicity testing for new food additives. The safety of all food additives must now be proven before they can be added to food. Yet most of the ingredients in foods have never been tested for carcinogenic properties! In fact, some of the substances generally regarded as safe—sugar and salt for example—have been demonstrated to cause cancer in animals. Unbelievable as this may sound, *if sugar and salt were discovered today, they would not pass the safety guidelines of the FDA, and they would never be approved as food additives.*

There are some foods you should avoid altogether, such as alfalfa sprouts and moldy foods. Dried alfalfa sprouts fed to monkeys caused an autoimmune disease similar to *Lupus erythematosus.* And be wary of any food that has come in contact with the soil and is stored in warm, moist conditions. Aflatoxin, a potent mold toxin, often contaminates peanuts and cereal grains, and causes liver cancer.

Dining Out

Choose restaurants carefully. There are a number of crucial considerations. Many progressive restaurants offer low-fat selections and will allow you to choose the cooking method. Pick restaurants that have a salad bar because you can often satisfy your cancer-slashing daily needs with one pass at a salad bar! Keep in mind, however, that blue cheese, ranch, and Caesar salad dressings are high in fat.

Eat Ethnic Cuisines

Most cancer-suppressing groups are found in ethnic cooking. Japanese and French diets were discussed in detail earlier. Add to your list restaurants and recipes for Italian, Indian, Thai, Mexican, Mediterranean, and Chinese cuisine. Ethnic dishes are excellent choices and offer large portions of steamed vegetables and rice in relation to meats. It's not unreasonable to request that your food be cooked with less soy sauce or salt. Don't skimp on Italian and Mediterranean pasta-based dishes made with generous amounts of garlic and onions. Order a salad or a baked potato in place of french fries. Always request that butter and other high-fat sauces be served on the side.

Choose exciting, spicy selections that use small amounts of meat, poultry, and seafood. Rather than eat a full meat-based portion, split a main course and eat a large portion of fruit, salad, vegetables, or rice.

Don't skimp on omelets at restaurants willing to make egg-white omelets. Egg white is protein-rich while the yolk is cholesterol-rich.

Substitute lemon juice in place of salad dressing, and always order your dressing on the side, and use it sparingly.

Reverse the order of courses. As an alternative ask the server to bring your main course first, followed by a salad, especially if you eat meat. Sip beverages (red wine is acceptable) and small amounts of water during the first twenty minutes of your meal; otherwise you will dilute digestive acids and digest the protein poorly. When you finish your salad, drink more water and finish your wine. This will serve to swell (hydrate) your proteins and help satisfy your appetite.

It is beneficial to split your dessert. Instead of gorging on an oversized fattening dessert, halve it and order mineral water to go with it. It's easy to pick desserts that are low in fat. If you eat pie, try not to eat much crust. As a rule eat fruit before sugar, and sugar before fat.

Daily Diet

How do you put all this together and structure a day around crushing cancer with your diet? Herculean efforts are not required to weave cancer-busting foods into your meals. It's simply a matter of selecting the right foods, some of which are most likely already in your diet.

The menu plan of the cancer-busting regimen is simple and straightforward:

- Combine fresh foods from the Super Eight Food Groups.
- Substantially reduce consumption of meat, seafood, and dairy products.
- Avoid processed food products such as instant potatoes, cake, frozen dinners, packaged lunch meats, bologna, and hot dogs. Many processed foods are high-calorie foods that provide *empty* calories (calories from sugar and fat) that have been stripped of cancer-busting agents.

It's easy to move from a meat-based diet to a low-fat, anticancer diet if you follow the three phases detailed here: Starter, Advanced, and Optimal Diet Plans. Even implementing one of these three phases will help you extinguish cancer.

- The Starter Diet Plan attempts to increase cancer-quelling agents and decrease dietary fat by reducing your intake of dairy, meat, poultry, and fish.
- The Advanced Diet Plan greatly increases cancer-suppressing foods and substitutes dairy with soy protein.
- The Optimal Diet Plan offers the greatest level of anticancer clout by including the highest consumption of Super Eight Food Groups and the lowest consumption of dairy, meat, poultry, and fish.

Since fat nourishes the growth of many cancers, reduction in dietary fats is the first accomplishment in the Starter plan. There are many easy, tasty ways to reduce intake of dietary fat:

- Use smaller amounts of fat and cooking oils for food preparation.
- Use less saturated fat.
- If you eat meat, choose a lean cut and free-range variety.
- For sandwiches, use mustard to replace mayonnaise.
- As stated before, use only sesame seed, olive, and macadamia nut oils for cooking. Employ low-fat alternatives, but

remember that "Lite" or "Lyte" does not necessarily mean less fat. Be a skeptical label reader.

A particularly good way to lessen fat is to cut down on consumption of meat, poultry, and dairy products. Preorder the vegetarian meal when on airline flights. Go easy on meat, but if you must eat meat, poultry, and eggs, then choose free-range varieties raised with the freedom of the range and that have not been given hormones or growth stimulants. If you do nothing else to reduce fat, do not eat meat at every meal. The evidence is clear that eating meat once a day is more than sufficient.

If you cannot remember the Super Eight Food Groups, then choose a rainbow of different colors of vegetables and fruits, and alternate among eating Italian, Mexican, Chinese, and Japanese foods.

Choose fruit more often. Great fruits for warding off cancer are cantaloupe, grapefruit, oranges, bananas, raspberries, strawberries, blueberries, pears, and apples. Give frozen fruits a chance since many freeze very well. And use more low-sugar fruit spreads.

Opt for whole grain cereals more often, and make selections such as whole wheat and rye breads, bran bagels or oat bran pancakes. Make the most out of using low-fat toppings on your pancakes (for example, applesauce with cinnamon and berries).

General Dietary Rules

Rely on cancer-deterring fruit juices, fruit juice mixed with club soda, or club soda with lime or lemon juice. Fresh fruit juices have more anticancer clout and are typical breakfast drinks. You can further boost their cancer-zapping power and make a meal out of drinks by blending soy products or low-fat yogurt together with your favorite fruits. Real brewed ginger ales are a great beverage.

Avoid cancer-inciting fried foods of any kind, such as sausage and bacon (you can sample but don't feast on them). Also avoid butter, whole milk, cream, eggs, creamy salads, processed luncheon meats, and high-fat cheeses such as Swiss, cheddar, and American cheese.

Rely on cancer-crippling four-bean chili, spicy burritos made of beans, rice, and cheese, pasta, rice-based dishes, and salads with beans or mixed dark greens. Also use plenty of vegetables such as green beans, broccoli, cauliflower, carrots, and celery.

Avoid splurging on meat-based selections. This does not mean don't eat meat at all, but select a rice-based dish with meat in it, or split a main course and have a generous salad.

Rely on rice and a variety of vegetable-based selections. Select combination dishes, such as chicken or tuna salad or shrimp with rice. Skip fatty buttered dressing and sprinkle with lemon and herbs. Or use a nonfat butter substitute. Shun high-fat condiments, instead top your baked potatoes with low-fat yogurt, chives, salsa, or low-fat cheese.

Starter Diet Plan Sample Menus

Starter Diet Plan—Breakfast (vegetarian)
    Bagel (oat bran, rye, wheat, sesame seed)
    Fresh-squeezed orange juice or whole orange
    Pink grapefruit (eat a whole one) with berries
    Italian Omelet
    Smokey snaps (a great alternative to bacon) or Glomorgan sausages

Starter Diet Plan—Lunch
    Chinese chicken salad
    Fruit salad with low-fat yogurt
    Lotus chicken
    Steamed rice with vegetables
    Green tea, fruit juice

Starter Diet Plan—Dinner
    Mexican-style fresh tomato pasta
    Curried chicken and spinach pasta salad
    Salad, including dark greens, carrots, and celery
    Cauliflower or broccoli soup
    Chocolate mint brownies
    Tea or red wine

See chapter 13 for recipes.

Snacks
For quick and easy snacks between meals, try eating fruits (like apples, oranges, peaches, or grapes) and raw vegetables (such as celery, carrots, and cucumber). You can buy bags of prewashed and peeled baby carrots and other vegetables in many stores.

Another great low-fat snack is plain air-popped popcorn, or popcorn cooked in a small amount of sesame oil. Packaged microwave popcorn contains a tremendous amount of fat. Instead of potato chips try low-fat alternatives like blue corn tortillas with salsa, or whole wheat squares with a small amount of parmesan cheese melted on top.

Great cancer combatants are nuts and seeds such as pumpkin seeds, flax seeds, sesame seeds, pistachio nuts, almonds, and walnuts. They make great snacks even though they're high in fat. You can effortlessly add nuts and seeds to your diet by sprinkling a handful on salads and by eating them as snacks. Licorice is another cancer-busting snack, but be sure to buy real licorice root extract. For dessert, try tofu ice cream, fresh fruit, Italian fruit gelato, and frozen fruit bars.

Advanced Diet Plan

The Advanced Diet Plan substitutes soy products for dairy. There are dozens of easy, tasty ways to include cancer-fighting soy:

- Add soy milk to your coffee or tea.
- Use soy milk in pancakes.
- Make a soy milk fruit shake.
- Add soy to stir fry dishes.
- Replace ricotta cheese with tofu in lasagna.
- Add soy protein to soups.

Soy comes in many forms, including tofu. Tofu's health benefits are too compelling to dismiss from your diet. Straight from the package tofu (which is made from soy milk) is bland, so most people don't like to eat it that way. But its ability to be transformed into something delicious is almost boundless. Silken tofu is white with a jellylike structure, so it falls apart easily. This makes silken tofu great to add to fruit shakes, cheesecake, or anything that needs a creamy texture. Since it easily falls apart, silken tofu is not good to grill, sauté, or fry. Regular tofu is a white slab that holds its shape when it is sliced or diced. It is available in three forms: soft, firm, or extra firm. The beauty of regular tofu is that it acts like a sponge, absorbing spices and flavors. Firm and extra firm tofu can be cooked like eggs, used in place of ricotta cheese in lasagna, added to soups, or grilled.

Soy milk is a liquid form of soy. It comes in vanilla, carob, and regular flavors. Soy milk can be used in place of milk in many recipes, and you can readily add soy milk to hot drinks like coffee, tea, or hot cocoa.

Soy flour can lend home-baked goods a moist texture and nutty flavor. This flour works well in cookies, pancakes, and muffins. It also makes a great substitute for eggs (1 tablespoon of soy flour mixed with 1 tablespoon of water replaces 1 egg). Soy flour baked goods brown faster, so use lower cooking temperatures and shorter baking times. The cooking possibilities for soy products are endless.

Advanced Diet Plan Sample Menus

Advanced Diet Plan—Breakfast
- Fruit shake with soy milk
- Fresh juice and fruits
- Coffee or tea with soy milk
- Cinnamon apple oat bran cereal
- Scrambled soy omelet with broccoli and cauliflower

Advanced Diet Plan—Lunch
- Fettuccine with broccoli and tomatoes
- Bean, rice, and cheese burrito with tomato based salsa or
- Italian ziti bake with onion, garlic, and tomato sauce
- Salad bar with fruit
- Ice tea with fresh lemon

Advanced Diet Plan—Dinner
    Spicy four bean chili
    Walnut pesto with acorn squash
    Stuffed peppers
    Tomato basil salad
    Baked potato with chives and low fat yogurt

See chapter 13 for recipes.

Optimal Diet Plan Sample Menus

Optimal Diet Plan—Breakfast
    Fresh citrus fruit (grapefruit or orange)
    Fruit shake with soy
    Oatmeal (not instant) with fresh berries and bananas
    Muesli pancakes with fresh fruit
    Tea with soy milk
    Grapefruit or orange juice

Optimal Diet Plan—Lunch
    Layered fruit salad
    Chinese noodle salad
    Mexican-style tomato pasta with garlic and onions
    Zesty tomato tofu soup

Optimal Diet Plan—Dinner
    Zucchini lasagna with soy
    Spaghetti squash stuffed with tomatoes
    Minestrone soup
    Mixed vegetables, green beans, almonds, and walnuts
    Garlic bread
    Red wine (two glasses at most)

See chapter 13 for recipes.

The Optimal Diet Plan provides the highest level of chemopre-vention since it is mostly a semi-vegetarian or plant-based diet. Ideally you should follow one of the cancer-blocking diet phases all the time. However, in our world of fast processed foods and dinner parties, few people can adhere to a specialized diet. So if you only deviate on weekends, you will still receive substantial anticancer benefits. By choosing a proper mixture of cancer-battering foods during the weekdays, you won't have to worry on the weekends.

Chapter Recap

- Complete protection requires the Super Eight Food Groups, not reliance on one miracle nutrient.
- The cancer-busting regimen, which is based on naturally occurring agents found in the Super Eight Food Groups from around the world, provides optimal cancer suppression.
- There are methods to prepare food that minimize formation of cancer-producing substances.
- A number of dietary agents protect against the toxic compounds formed by grilling or charbroiling food.

Cancer-Busting Vitamins

Something is amiss in the controversy surrounding vitamin supplements. Some say vitamin supplements are completely unnecessary, while many vitamin guzzlers swear by them. If you followed the Cancer-Busting Regimen and lived in an ideal world then you would not need vitamin supplements. Unfortunately, in today's world no one lives pollution-free, and many of us are relying on a Western diet low in cancer-curbing agents. When in doubt, take vitamin supplements.

Man cannot live by bread alone.

—Deuteronomy 8:3

After all, vitamins are essential nutrients. Without them disease and premature death can occur. Using vitamins is a major anticancer defense.

How Do Vitamins Protect?

As we learned earlier, enzymes are highly specialized proteins that accelerate chemical reactions taking place in the body. Without these speeded-up chemical reactions, life as we humans know it would be impossible. Most enzymes require cofactors to work efficiently, such as water-soluble vitamins and minerals. The human body can make proteins, but vitamin cofactors must be obtained from the diet.

For instance, vitamin B6 is needed in over half of the body's reactions involving enzymes, while folic acid is required for the activity of enzymes involved in making DNA.

When the enzyme has enough cofactor (or vitamin), additional amounts of that cofactor do nothing to increase enzyme activity. This has led researchers to widely conclude that a higher intake of vitamins is wasteful and serves no useful purpose. But as more discoveries are made concerning other features, such as the anticancer action of vitamins, this position is being reconsidered. For example, vitamins stymie formation of cancer-causing chemicals, and many have potent antioxidant activity (for instance vitamins C, E, and beta carotene).

Some vitamins are linked to reduced cancer risk and also have a low toxicity, even when taken 100 to 1,000 times over the Recommended Daily Dietary Allowances (RDA). Again, these include C, E, folic acid, and beta carotene. Research continues to suggest that the RDA may not provide optimal health benefits under all circumstances. Many people have health problems, risky lifestyles, or reside in extremely polluted environments, so their intake of vitamins definitely should exceed the RDA.

Good Times to Exceed the RDA for Vitamins

- When using pain killing-drugs
- While smoking cigarettes or using tobacco
- If using oral contraceptives
- During disorders of the digestive tract
- During laxative use
- While ingesting caffeine drinks
- When drinking alcoholic beverages
- When exposed to pollutants
- If chemical exposure occurs at work
- If your diet is inadequate
- If you need X-rays

Special Vitamin Needs

Certain life styles and particular times of life may require you to boost your intake of vitamins.

Tobacco smoking is associated with an increased risk of cancer, heart disease, and chronic lung disease (see chapter 11). It's also true that smokers have low levels of key antioxidant vitamins. For example, smokers tend to have much lower levels of vitamin C, beta carotene, and vitamin B6 in their blood. Male smokers not only have lower vitamin C levels, but show increased damage to their sperm. In any case, smokers clearly have an increased demand for vitamin C. They have also been shown to have much lower levels of vitamin E in their lungs than nonsmokers. So reduced vitamin levels may contribute to some of the health risks associated with smoking.

Weight-reducing diets that restrict whole categories of food can seriously affect vitamin status. For instance, diets that eliminate all animal foods will provide only meager amounts of vitamin B12. Skipping meals and dieting result in skimpy vitamin intake. Hence it is almost impossible to meet all of your vitamin requirements while on a weight-reducing diet unless you take supplements.

Medications can also cause mayhem, either by increasing the body's demand for more vitamins, or by blocking absorption of vitamins. The use of oral contraceptives is associated with decreased levels of beta carotene, vitamin B6, vitamin C, and folic acid. Many common medications, including antibiotics and antacids, are known to interfere with the uptake of vitamins. Both aspirin and antiepilepsy drugs can inhibit the uptake of folic acid, and when taken daily these drugs can cause vitamin deficiencies.

A regular intake of alcohol alters the activity of vitamin D and is associated with low blood levels of beta carotene, folic acid, thiamin, and vitamin B6. Steady use of alcohol will often cause extremely low liver stores of vitamin A. Alcohol has also been shown to hinder absorption of vitamin C.

In adolescence, which is a period of rapid growth, vitamin demands are often not met because of poor eating habits. Nutritional studies reveal folic acid to be deficient in about half of otherwise healthy teenage girls. Today more teens are overweight, with poor nutrition resulting from widespread attempts at dieting for weight reduction.

Pregnancy is a period of increased vitamin demand. Balanced nutrition is extremely critical during the first trimester of pregnancy. Even with seemingly normal, healthy pregnancies, almost one fourth of women are deficient in at least one essential vitamin at the time of childbirth.

In old age people often are short of vitamins. This may be due to inadequate diet, dental conditions, or chronic illness. For example, the ability to digest and absorb vitamins is often reduced in older people. One study revealed that the elderly have less ability to obtain folic acid from foods and to digest time-release vitamins.

Essential Vitamins

The most vital anticancer vitamins are A, beta carotene, E, C, folic acid, niacin, B6, and B12.

Vitamin A

Numerous studies show that vitamin A plays a critical role in reproduction, the growth of skin, and vision. Vitamin A is mainly stored in the liver. In people with well-balanced diets, enough vitamin A is stored to last many months. The first sign of vitamin A deficiency is night blindness; if this deficiency continues, it can lead to irreversible blindness.

HEALTH BENEFITS OF VITAMIN A

reduces risk of breast, lung, throat, and oral cancers

increases immune response

protects tobacco chewers from oral cancer

helps maintain skin

decreases the possibility of cancer's reoccurrence

Rich dietary sources of vitamin A include dairy products, eggs, and vegetables like asparagus, broccoli, carrots, peas, and pumpkin. Beta carotene, which is found in deep-yellow and dark-green vegetables, can be converted to vitamin A during digestion.

The RDA of vitamin A for adults is 5,000 IU.

Vitamin A may prevent cancer in several ways. It is well known that vitamin A fosters growth and maintains your surface cells or *epithelial* tissues, which is where many cancers arise. Vitamin A also plays a critical role in the immune system by hindering tumor cell growth.

Pneumonia and frequent infections in animals are linked with low levels of vitamin A. A short supply of vitamin A is believed to reduce resistance to infection by hampering the normal growth and production of mucus-secreting cells. It is probable that vitamin A is quite important for proper immune system functioning, since it significantly increases the ability of human immune cells to kill tumors.

Vitamin A is more toxic than other vitamins discussed in this chapter. Therefore, it is not advised to significantly increase your intake of this vitamin beyond the RDA. This is especially true for pregnant women. Vitamin A in very large doses is known to cause birth defects in many animals.

Beta carotene

Beta carotene is part of a family of plant pigments that result in the yellow, orange, and red colors of fruits and vegetables. Though over

600 carotenoids have been identified in nature, beta carotene is one of the most abundant carotenoids found in human foods. As such, it plays an important role in cancer prevention. Beta carotene is converted into vitamin A, and many believe that its protective actions are based on its conversion into this vitamin.

However, several lines of evidence are now applauding beta carotene's effectiveness against cancer. Beta carotene has the ability to reduce the toxicity of an active form of oxygen (so-called *singlet oxygen*). Singlet oxygen, which is capable of damaging tissues, is highly reactive and turns out to be an important element in light-sensitive skin disorders. Beta carotene is the most effective naturally occurring agent that is able to hinder the toxicity from singlet oxygen. By acting as an antioxidant and blocking mutagenic activity, beta carotene reduces the risk of cancer.

A careful survey shows that beta carotene can enhance immune function, including suppression of tumors. Several animal studies have also shown immune function improvement following intake of beta carotene.

Beta carotene may provide a counteroffensive for people who smoke, since levels of beta carotene are lower in smokers than in nonsmokers. When smokers take the same amount of beta carotene as nonsmokers, they still end up with lower blood levels of that vitamin, suggesting that smokers have a greater need for beta carotene and should take larger amounts.

Observers have noted that beta carotene seems to be its most potent against lung cancer. There is also a strong relationship between low intake of beta carotene and increased rates for cervix, throat, digestive tract, lung, oral, and stomach cancers. What's more, beta carotene seems to protect against UV-induced skin cancer. And a high dietary intake of beta carotene and green vegetables have been found to contribute to decreased risk of developing breast cancer.

Finally, people with low beta carotene levels have about a six times greater chance of developing vision-impairing cataracts. This is surprising since the lens of the eye contains very little beta carotene. Clouding in the lens of the eye that leads to formation of cataracts is

HEALTH BENEFITS OF BETA CAROTENE

contains antioxidant properties

improves the immune system

protects in light sensitive-skin disorders

protects from cancer

reduces lung, cervix, stomach, throat, endometrial, breast, oral cancers

protects from the effects of tobacco

protects from cataracts in the eye

linked to oxidative conditions. So it is believed that beta carotene protects from cataracts by reducing the overall oxidative reactions in the body, thus indirectly sparing the lens.

Beta carotene is relatively nontoxic. Though it is converted into vitamin A, the body only converts what is needed; therefore, higher intakes of beta carotene do not lead to high levels of vitamin A. Excessive intake of beta carotene can cause a yellow skin coloring, which is reversible and apparently harmless. The RDA for adults is 50 IU.

Vitamin E

Vitamin E (tocopherol) is an essential vitamin. Alpha-tocopherol is the most biologically friendly form of vitamin E, and it is especially suited to defend cell membranes. Cell membranes are largely composed of polyunsaturated fats, and these are easily oxidized (similar to the process that turns butter rancid). So one of the prime functions of vitamin E is to preserve membranes from this rancidity. Vitamin E is a vital antioxidant, which also plays a crucial role in the immune system, inhibits formation of mutagens, and is involved in the repair of membranes and DNA.

Vitamin E is stored mainly in fat tissue, the liver, and muscles, although it has been shown to be stored in all tissues when the intake is high.

Some of the richest sources of vitamin E are wheat germ oil, brans and legumes, vegetable oils, nuts, seeds, and green plants. The adult RDA of vitamin E is 30 IU.

HEALTH BENEFITS OF VITAMIN E

enhances immune system

may prevent digestive tract, lung, breast, prostate, and throat cancer

protects from neurological disorders

is involved in DNA repair

may prevent heart disease—vitamin E is a factor in heart disease

may prevent strokes

decreases platelet aggregation and adhesion, which is critical for preventing strokes

has antioxidant properties

blocks nitrosamine formation

is involved in cell membrane repair

As we learned previously, nitrosamines that damage DNA and cause cancer are normally formed in the body from nitrates and nitrites present in foods and even cigarette smoke. Vitamin E suppresses the conversion of these cancer-causing nitrosamines. A sensible amount of vitamins C and E (400 mg/day) can restrict the amount of mutagenic compounds (like nitrosamines) in the digestive tract by 75 percent. Time after time studies show that individuals with low vitamin E intake are much more prone to cancers of the lung, breast, digestive tract, and throat.

When a blood vessel is severed, small corpuscles called platelets (which are central to the clotting process) stick to the injured site, then clump together. During this clumping process the platelets release chemical signals that further increase clumping, eventually stopping the flow of blood. Of course, this clumping process is vital to our survival. There is a dark side to this process, however. When the platelet response becomes exaggerated, then clumping occurs too easily, and the result of that may be a heart attack or stroke. In any case, this sequence of platelet clumping can contribute to development of heart disease. The good news is that vitamin E has been shown to keep platelet response in check. It's important to keep in mind, though, that vitamin E content in platelets declines with age.

Like beta carotene, vitamin E has been shown to reduce the incidence of cataracts. In general, antioxidants protect against cataract formation in humans. Therefore, by combining high vitamin E intake with beta carotene and vitamin C, you can significantly decrease the possibility of your developing cataracts.

Vitamin E deficiencies are linked with neurological disorders like Alzheimer's and Parkinson's disease. It is believed that vitamin E stabilizes and protects membranes through its actions as an antioxidant. In fact, nervous tissue such as that found in the brain is known to be particularly susceptible to oxidative damage. Finally, environmental pollutants also clearly play a role in nervous system diseases, and vitamin E seems to help in the prevention.

Precautions: Even taken at very high levels, vitamin E has few toxic side effects. Vitamin E can increase blood clotting time in individuals with certain diseases or with vitamin K deficiencies. Individuals who are taking blood thinning drugs (anticoagulants) should be careful of high vitamin E intake.

Vitamin C

Vitamin C is an antioxidant, and it limits the activity of free radicals, protecting cell membranes and other important structures.

Rich dietary sources of vitamin C include citrus fruits, cruciferous vegetables, peppers, and potatoes.

The RDA of vitamin C in adults is 60 milligrams.

Vitamin C is necessary for making collagen, the most common protein in the body. Collagen is part of the supporting structure of skin, cartilage, tendons, ligaments, bones, teeth, and blood vessels. Without plenty of vitamin C, collagen that is formed is weak, easily degraded, and is more susceptible to tumor invasion.

As an antioxidant, vitamin C protects DNA from free radical damage and from mutagens. For instance, vitamin C reduces harmful genetic damage in workers who have been exposed to DNA-damaging chemicals.

In addition to acting as an antioxidant, vitamin C may prevent cancer by blocking the formation of nitrosamines. In human studies, vitamin C significantly limited levels of nitrosamines. Vitamin C also hinders the mutagenic potential of gastric juice.

So vitamin C is likely to prevent cancer by acting as an antioxidant, by restricting the formation of nitrosamines and mutagens, by enhancing the immune system, and by promoting the detoxification of toxic chemicals. For example, high vitamin C intake is associated with fewer disorders of the digestive tract, such as oral, throat, stomach, colon, and rectal cancers. Vitamin C may also protect against lung, cervix, and pancreatic cancers. People with a high risk of throat cancer consume far less vitamin C and fewer fresh fruits and vegetables than those with a low risk.

If stomach cancer is the final product of a long-term siege on the stomach lining (and it is believed that it is), then ulcers are early warning signals. In order to reduce nitrosamine levels and the mutagenic activity of stomach juices as well, take 1 gram of vitamin C each day. Because generation of nitrosamines in the stomach probably plays a critical role in stomach cancer, it is vital to have plenty of vitamin C present at exactly the same time as you eat high nitrite/nitrate foods (such as processed meats).

HEALTH BENEFITS OF VITAMIN C

reduces cancer risk—foods rich in vitamin C may protect against oral, throat, stomach, colon, rectal, lung, cervix, and pancreatic cancer

reduces risk of stroke

acts as an antioxidant

blocks formation of cancer-causing chemicals like nitrosamines

influences stronger bone growth

improves wound healing

improves cardiovascular health

may lower blood pressure

prevents cataract formation

blocks formation of fecal mutagens

enhances clearance of toxic chemicals in the liver

reduces the toxicity of some pollutants like pesticides, heavy metals, hydrocarbons, ozone, carbon monoxide

enhances immune system functions

What about the other areas of protection offered by vitamin C? It is believed that vitamin C stimulates the immune system by enhancing the function of white blood cells. Vitamin C may also boost resistance to infection by promoting formation of stronger collagen, which in turn provides a better barrier against bacteria, viruses, and tumor cells.

Since vitamin C is necessary for proper collagen formation, antioxidant protection, and may encourage the burning of fat, it may also protect from heart disease. A major risk factor for heart disease is high blood pressure. And blood pressure levels are higher in those who take in very little vitamin C. Also, like vitamin E, vitamin C inhibits platelet aggregation and adhesion, which is a critical stage in the development of heart disease.

And what about strokes? Strokes that afflict brain function are linked to blood vessel damage, free radical activity, atherosclerosis, and high blood pressure. Since vitamin C influences all of these processes, it is likely that it lowers the risk of stroke.

Finally, vitamin C supplements protect from cataract risk. It is well known that ultraviolet light promotes cataract formation, and that cataracts are more common in countries with strong sunlight exposure. In nutritional studies, subjects who did not take vitamin C (300 to 600 mg/day) had four times higher risk of developing cataracts.

Vitamin C is a relatively nontoxic vitamin. There are few toxic side effects, even when taken in extreme doses. One side effect is diarrhea. Another concern is that vitamin C is partially converted into oxalates, which are major components of kidney stones. However, many studies have shown that high doses of vitamin C do not cause kidney stones. It may be prudent for people who have a tendency to form kidney stones, or who have kidney disease, to limit their intake of vitamin C.

Folic Acid

Folic acid is a critical component of several important enzymes that are required for the manufacture of nucleic acids (like DNA) and for utilization of some amino acids. Folic acid deficiency results in decreased production of deoxyribonucleic acid (DNA), ribonucleic acid (RNA), and certain proteins. Folic acid is also required for proper DNA repair, which is critical in preventing the progression of cancer.

Good food sources of folic acid are dark green leafy vegetables, lentils, soybeans, nuts, beans, fresh fruits and vegetables, and yeast.

The RDA of folic acid for adults is 400 micrograms. For pregnant women the RDA is 800 micrograms.

Folic acid demands are greatest during growth phases. Therefore it is not surprising that the risk of deficiency is highest in infants, adolescents, and pregnant women. During pregnancy there is an increased need for folic acid, due to the rapid growth of the developing infant. Sufficient folic acid is extremely critical for proper infant growth during pregnancy. Early in pregnancy during the closure of the neural tube (which matures into the spinal cord), a lack of folic acid will result in neural tube defects. Cleft palate and cleft lip are birth defects also linked to low folic acid in the mother's diet.

HEALTH BENEFITS OF FOLIC ACID

prevents neural tube and cleft palate defects

required for DNA manufacture and repair

critical for a healthy heart and vessels

may reduce risk of cancers of the uterus, cervix, intestine, colon, and lungs

may reduce risk of chromosome defects

Don't skimp on folic acid since its intake combats colon, intestinal, and cervical cancer. Diets meager in folic acid have been associated with precancerous conditions in the uterus, cervix, and intestine. Women with existing cervical cancer have lower folic acid levels than those without cancer.

Precancer cells are often seen years before full-blown cancer. Folic acid intake in smokers has been shown to prevent formation of precancer cells in the lung.

Folic acid is required to convert the amino acid homocysteine to methionine, a conversion that is critical for a healthy heart. If there is too little folic acid, homocysteine will build up. High levels of homocysteine are believed to cause heart disease.

Folic acid is relatively nontoxic and safe, even when intake is very high. Alcohol, drugs to control convulsions, and oral contraceptives are known to interfere with, or lower, folic acid levels.

Niacin

Niacin (vitamin B3 or nicotinic acid) is another critical cofactor in a number of different processes, but most notably energy production.

Niacin is found in many foods like whole grains and peanuts.

The RDA of niacin is 20 milligrams for adults.

High doses of niacin in the form of nicotinic acid have been used to treat people with high cholesterol. Nicotinic acid decreases the so-called "bad" or LDL cholesterol (low-density lipoprotein cholesterol) and enhances the healthy HDL cholesterol (high density lipoprotein cholesterol). A study that followed men after they suffered their first heart attack revealed that those who received niacin supplements had a death rate 11 percent lower than those who did not take niacin.

Many people who take in high doses of nicotinic acid will experience temporary skin flushing. This flushing of the skin is not an adverse reaction, and many people develop a tolerance over time. The niacinamide form of niacin that is typically found in vitamin pills does not cause skin flushing, yet neither does it have the fat (lipid) lowering effect of nicotinic acid.

HEALTH BENEFITS OF VITAMIN B12

prevents cancer

enhances immune system

prevents heart disease

Vitamins B12 and B6

Vitamin B12 is essential for the enzymes involved in the manufacture of amino acids, fatty acids, and DNA. Vitamin B12 is also required for the function of folic acid. A B12 deficiency can lead to irreversible nervous system damage.

Vitamin B12 is found almost exclusively in foods of animal origin. It is primarily stored in the liver.

The RDA of vitamin B12 for adults is 6 micrograms.

Vitamin B6 is a cofactor in over 100 enzyme reactions, and it is vital for DNA repair and cardiac health.

The RDA of vitamin B6 for adults is 2 milligrams.

Heavy smokers who have supplemented with both vitamin B12 and folic acid have shown remarkable decreases in precancer cells, compared to smokers not given these vitamins. What's more, studies with animals suggest that vitamin B12 may suppress tumor cell growth.

Earlier we learned that folic acid is critical for the conversion of homocysteine to methionine. Vitamin B6 and B12 are required for this transformation also (as are magnesium and biotin).

It is not surprising that if there is a deficiency in either vitamin B6 or B12, homocysteine will accumulate. When homocysteine levels rise, this causes damage to the interior of vessels (or arteriosclerosis), and it may increase the risk of heart disease. People at high risk for heart disease have elevated levels of homocysteine.

There are very few side effects for vitamin B12, even with high doses in excess of the RDA.

Chapter Recap

- Vitamins A, C, E, beta carotene, and folic acid are another line of chemopreventive defense and have been consistently associated with reduced cancer risks.
- Vitamins have additional benefits, including enhancing immune system function and preventing heart disease, cataracts, birth defects, and stroke.
- Be careful with high intakes of vitamin A. On the other hand, vitamins C, E, beta carotene, and folic acid are relatively nontoxic and can be well tolerated by most people even at very high intakes.

The Cancer Conquering Female: Defeating Breast Cancer and Other Female Cancers

Women have been at risk for breast cancer throughout human history. The first record of breast cancer was probably made by the Egyptians, yet in ancient times few Egyptian women seem to have died of the disease. In modern times, however, breast cancer has taken on a different guise. Just thirty-five years ago American women had a one-in-twenty chance of getting breast cancer. Today the chances are almost three in twenty. Why is this?

> The vast majority of breast cancers are not genetic ones. Only about 10 percent of breast cancers have that family history behind them.
>
> —Marlys Schuh, surgical oncologist

Social Status and Cancer

Statistics continue to bear out a surprising trend that has been known for over a century: The higher a woman's social status, the more apt she is to get breast cancer. Some presumed reasons for this are that wealthy women tend to have fewer children, later in life. They breastfeed less, and they eat rich, Western diets. But why are lifestyle factors so crucial to breast cancer rates? It appears that the longer a woman's fertile lifespan is (in other words, the greater the number of menstrual cycles she goes through during her life), the more prone she is to breast cancer.

Until 1960 the death rate for breast cancer in Japan was only one-sixth that of the Western world. One of the main reasons given for this is that, until the 1960s, the average Japanese woman started menstruating later than American women—about age sixteen, as opposed to age twelve or thirteen for Americans.

Since 1960 Japanese women have suffered from a 36 percent increase in breast cancer deaths, the highest increase in the world. During the same time period, the age of onset of menstruation dropped from an average age of sixteen to fourteen years old. This earlier puberty, which sets the stage for breast cancer, has been directly related to an increased intake of Western foods.

Some argue that breast cancer is not caused by rich fatty foods. Rather it is caused by what the fat is laden with, and that includes environmental chemicals such as PCBs, DDT, and dioxin. These chemicals are known to mimic estrogen activity. And, as will soon be explained, increased estrogen activity results in more risk of breast cancer.

What sensible steps can a woman take to stem the risk of breast cancer? Most women do not realize that breast cancer is a preventable disease. Countless lives can be saved with a proper anticancer diet.

In different parts of the world, the incidence of breast cancer varies dramatically. Breast cancer (which is actually a collection of different cancers) is far more common in North America and Western Europe than in South and Central America, Greenland, and much of Asia. Since breast cancer is high in North America and Europe, and notably lower in Greenland and Japan, it seems more than likely that diet and environmental factors are at work.

To fully address the role that diet and environment play, let us look at the basic breast structure, and also at how estrogen is linked to breast cancer.

At the cellular level a normal breast is a collection of mostly fatty tissue with scattered milk-producing glands and an orderly series of slender, branching ducts channeling to the nipple. Breast milk is produced in bulbous glands known as lobules.

Breast cancer that begins in the lobules (lobular carcinoma) is not common and only accounts for 10 percent of all breast cancers. Up to 90 percent of breast cancer arises in the ducts (ductal carcinoma). Since the ducts, or ductile areas, of the breast are exquisitely influenced by hormonal activity, it's no wonder that most breast cancer arises there.

Menstrual Cycles

Evidence is compelling that the sex hormone estrogen can manipulate the development, and the invasiveness, of breast cancer. Estrogen and progesterone not only stimulate the growth of mammary glands and ducts, but normal monthly cell cycling makes the breasts vulnerable to cancer. When women experience tenderness in their breasts each month, it is due to the fact that estrogen is stimulating the breast cells to divide. During the first part of the twenty-eight-day menstrual cycle, estrogen levels sharply increase, then they fall back to normal

BREAST CANCER	
TYPE	FREQUENCY
Scirrhous Carcinoma[1]	75 percent
Medullary Carcinoma	5–10 percent
Mucinous Carcinoma	<5 percent
Intraductal Carcinoma[2]	5 percent
Lobular Carcinoma[3]	10 perecent

[1] Note that scirrhous, medullary, mucinous and intraductal are all considered ductal types of breast cancer.
[2] Noninvasive, however over time it will invade.
[3] Invasive

levels. The harm comes from normal estrogen levels ebbing and flowing over decades of menstruation, from puberty to menopause. The longer women are exposed to high estrogen levels, the more apt they are to get breast cancer.

Estrogen levels are at their highest just before ovulation, which usually occurs at mid-cycle, or fourteen days, It is known that breast cells divide more rapidly in the last fourteen days of each cycle. It is also known that dividing cells are more apt to damage DNA, ultimately increasing the risk of cancer.

In recent studies women who had shorter menstrual cycles had about twice the risk of breast cancer than women with a 28-day cycle. Similarly, women with longer-than-average menstrual cycles also had twice the risk of breast cancer. It is the extremes in cycle lengths that boost women's chance of getting breast cancer.

MENSTRUAL CYCLE		
PHASE	ACTIVITY	DAYS IN CYCLE
follicular phase (early)	menstruation begins	1–5
follicular phase (late)	egg develops into follicle[1]	6–13
ovulation	egg is released from ovary	Day 14
luteal phase	lining of uterus develops	15–28

[1] A follicle is a cellular mass containing an egg in the ovary.

Pregnancy

Women who bear children at a young age defuse the early onset of breast cancer. For unknown reasons pregnancy and lactation alter the breast tissues, making them less vulnerable to cancer.

RISK FACTORS FOR BREAST CANCER

age at first pregnancy—over 30

not nursing newborn—the longer the period of nursing, the greater the protection

having no children

early puberty—Western, rich diets favor early puberty or late menopause

use of oral contraceptives—raises risk slightly

estrogen supplements—for 6 years or more

obesity—adult obesity favors later menopause and increased breast cancer risk

Western diet—in particular, beef, pork, dairy products, fried potatoes, and cheese

alcohol

lack of exercise—women who exercise more than 15 hours per week were 60 percent less likely to have breast cancer; strenuous physical activity may also delay the onset of menstruation

radiation exposure

postmenopausal women with abdominal fatness

For example, a recent study showed that mothers who breastfeed have a 20 percent lower risk of contracting breast cancer, and that young mothers get the most anticancer benefits from breast feeding. Mothers aged nineteen or younger who nurse their infants for a period of six months reduce their risk of premenopausal breast cancer by 50 percent. Women who nursed for shorter periods still had significant protection. But researchers are perplexed because the protection gained is only in cancers that strike before menopause. For undiscovered reasons, breastfeeding has no impact on reducing the risk of breast cancer occurring after menopause.

These studies illustrate that hormone levels are critical in the development of breast cancer. Estrogen exerts many powerful influences, including changes in breast structure, cell membrane structure, and even changes in the immune system.

Understanding the role estrogen plays in the female life cycle can help you guard against breast cancer.

Diet to Prevent Breast Cancer

It's going to take researchers a long time to unravel the precise mechanisms of breast cancer. The exact sequence and order of events that may begin with fatty food to emergence of an aggressive cancer has not been pinpointed. Many of the risk factors for breast cancer are known, however. Some of the leading culprits are often beyond an individual's control, such as early menstruation, a family history of breast cancer, childbearing after age thirty, and late menopause. But several dietary elements seem to overpower breast cancer, primarily fiber, soy products, carotenoids, and cruciferous vegetables.

It is believed that breast cancer takes anywhere from three to thirty years to arise. So it is critical to receive cancer-quelling agents during this time frame. The practice of eating to beat cancer is a vital way to stop breast cancer in its tracks. The prevention meal plan against breast cancer encourages the use of the following foods:

- Soybean protein (soya and soy products—soy milk, tofu)
- Cruciferous vegetables (watercress, broccoli, cauliflower, brussels sprouts, mustard greens, collard, kale, Chinese cabbage)
- Protease inhibitors (seeds, nuts, legumes, beans, squash zucchini, rice, barley, rye, oats, cucumber seeds, potatoes)
- Fibers and lignans (plant fibers)
- Estrogen-lowering foods (legumes, whole grains, berries, broccoli, brussels sprouts)
- Vitamins and minerals (vitamins D, E, beta carotene, and selenium)
- Omega-3 fat foods (seafood, fish, flaxseed)
- Miscellaneous (green tea, licorice, melatonin, and enteric-coated aspirin)

You should also be careful to avoid:

- High-fat diets
- High animal-protein diets
- Safflower oil, corn oil, sunflower oil and cottonseed oil
- Dairy products
- Excess alcoholic beverages (red wine is okay in moderation)

Fat

There is considerable controversy surrounding the precise dietary components that might be responsible for encouraging breast cancer. The high fat/high risk theory was championed in the 1960s, supported by statistics reflecting high rates of breast cancer in countries where high amounts of fat are consumed. Western diets typically are 40 percent fat, while Asian diets at that time had only 15 percent fat.

In present-day Japan, where American-style fast food restaurants have been rapidly replacing traditional offerings of fish, rice, and vegetables, breast cancer has become more prevalent (although it is still less common than in the U.S.) Between 1965 and 1985, breast cancer in Japan increased by 50 percent! At the same time fat consumption rose dramatically. In 1955, the average Japanese woman consumed 6.5 grams of fat per day. In 1987, she ate four times that much: 28 grams per day.

In Japan there has also been a gradual increase in consumption of red meat. Many studies have connected this shift toward a Western-style diet with Japan's pronounced increase in breast cancer. Japanese who have migrated to Hawaii, and their subsequent generations, also show boosts in rates of breast cancer. Similar results appear in migration studies of Chinese and Polish women, whose subsequent generations living in the United States have escalating breast cancer rates.

Another interesting angle in the high fat/high risk theory is the effect low fat diets have on women who have already developed breast cancer and have been treated for it. Unexpectedly, it has been found that low-fat diets may quell the risk of reoccurrence in this group. In fact the typical Japanese breast cancer patient has a much better survival rate than her American counterpart. But American women with breast cancer avoid reoccurrence more often when they are on low-fat diets.

Recently a number of studies have contradicted the association between high fat diets and breast cancer. These scientists agree that breast cancer is more directly related to estrogen levels, which are directly and indirectly affected by excess dietary fats. In any case it remains a good idea to cut down on dietary fat, since many cancers (including melanoma, skin, liver, colon, rectal, and pancreatic cancers) are associated with high-fat diets.

The association between total fat consumption and breast cancer is consistent. Positive correlations with breast cancer have been shown among total calories, meat, sugar, and fatty foods. Negative correlations are shown with cereal, beans, rice, and maize.

Fat and Estrogen

It is not surprising that there are dozens of studies discussing the role of dietary fat on estrogen levels and the related development of breast cancer. Countries with diets high in fat have a skyrocketing incidence of breast cancer, compared to much lower statistics for countries consuming low-fat diets.

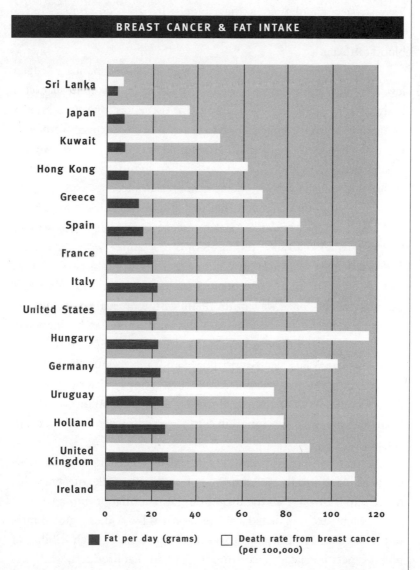

BREAST CANCER & FAT INTAKE

Fat per day (grams)   Death rate from breast cancer (per 100,000)

Figure 8

Fat is clearly a major culprit in fixing the amount of estrogen circulating in the blood, either by affecting the way a woman's body disposes of estrogen or by regulating the actual quantity of estrogen secreted. Women who eat meat with high levels of animal fat tend to reabsorb circulating estrogen rather than excrete it. On the other hand, vegetarian women tend to excrete more estrogen and have significantly less estrogen circulating in their blood. It has been shown that a woman who curbs her fat intake by 25 percent will reduce her levels of blood estrogen.

The fat stores in overweight women also enhance estrogen levels. Even after menopause, when estrogen levels should drop, excess body fat perpetuates estrogen supply. Fat tissue has long been known as a major source of lingering estrogen in postmenopausal women. If those women have significant abdominal fat, they have a twofold greater risk of developing breast cancer than slimmer women. Obesity is clearly associated with an increase in breast cancer.

The amount of fat in a diet may not be as critically important as the type of fat. Greenland, Alaska, and even Japan (in comparison to the continental U.S.) have few cases of breast cancer, which may have to do with higher consumption of omega-3 fats found in flaxseed, fish, and seafood. The most concentrated sources are found in cold water fish like halibut. Since we cannot manufacture omega-3 fats, they are essential to human diets. Omega-3 fats functioning as hormonelike derivatives play key roles as formidable deterrents to heart disease.

Omega-3 fats also seem to have anticancer clout. Studies have shown that mammary tumors in rodents regressed when omega-3 fats from fish oil were consumed. However, the typical American diet is laden with omega-6 fats, found in cottonseed, safflower, sunflower, and corn oils.

Nearly all tumor promoters stimulate the generation of arachidonic acid and products. Found in animal products like meat, arachidonic acid is involved in the promotion of mammary tumors.

Many exciting facts have been learned by studying global rates of breast cancer. In Moscow it was determined that a high liability of breast cancer is related to consumption of animal products, while less danger was associated with a high intake of fruits and vegetables.

Similar results were found in a Canadian study which showed that increasing consumption of fat in the form of beef, pork, butter, and fat-rich desserts leads to increased cancer risk. Another study among Chinese women living in Singapore found a reduced chance of cancer with high intakes of soy protein, beta carotene, and polyunsaturated fats.

A collective analysis of twelve human studies showed a direct association between the danger of breast cancer and intake of saturated fat. A decreased risk was found in diets rich in fruits, vegetables and vitamin C.

The National Cancer Institute has reported that women whose diets include large amounts of fruits, vegetables, and olive oil are more likely to arrest breast cancer. Olive oil itself may have cancer-blocking effects. An omega-9 monounsaturated fat, olive oil does not seem to have the tumor-promoting effects of omega-6 fats.

Estrogen

What you eat not only influences the levels of estrogen in your blood, but diet also alters the way your system handles sex hormones like estrogen.

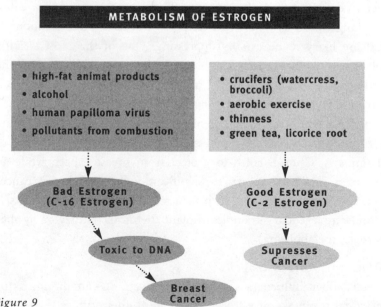

METABOLISM OF ESTROGEN

- high-fat animal products
- alcohol
- human papilloma virus
- pollutants from combustion

- crupeers (watercress, broccoli)
- aerobic exercise
- thinness
- green tea, licorice root

Bad Estrogen
(C-16 Estrogen)

Good Estrogen
(C-2 Estrogen)

Toxic to DNA

Supresses Cancer

Breast Cancer

Figure 9

Nature has provided two steps in estrogen metabolism that are pivotal concerning breast cancer. These are C-2 and C-16 alpha hydroxylation. Liver enzymes convert estrogen into both a so-called 2 hydroxy and a 16 hydroxy form. The C-16 form is the cancer-inciting villain of this pathway because it will fervently bind to proteins and pulverize DNA. In contrast, the C-2 form is the good form, acting as a potent cancer suppresser and antiestrogenic.

The C-2 avenue is accessible to everyone, but it is keenly tied to drug or dietary control. Thinness in a woman will boost the favorable C-2 pathway, while an obese state nullifies that pathway. Aerobic exercise also elevated the preferred C-2 pathway, thus cutting the odds of cancer.

The more abundant the C-2 pathway, the more cancer-curbing results are seen for breast cancer, uterine cancer, and fibrocystic breast disease. Fibrocystic breast disease is the most common disorder of the female breast, afflicting 50 percent of adult women. It is characterized by numerous small cysts, or isolated cysts, that respond to stimulatory changes from the menstrual cycle.

Dietary vegetables also influence the C-2 pathway. Landmark studies have discovered that cruciferous vegetables are a formidable dietary deterrent to breast cancer, and offer protection against colon and lung cancer as well. Crucifers possess at least three compounds that are likely to be cancer suppressing. One of the most striking substances is the indole-3-carbinol, which powerfully boosts the estrogen C-2 pathway. Green tea and licorice root have also been shown to favor the cancer-zapping C-2 pathway.

Certain plant chemicals may forcibly stifle cancer by altering hormone metabolism. A recent study showed that large intakes of vitamins A, C, or E failed to protect from breast cancer, while an increased intake of vegetables significantly deterred breast cancer risk. Cruciferous vegetables such as broccoli, cauliflower, and brussels sprouts are legendary examples of plant chemicals that favorably alter estrogen metabolism.

Fiber and Anti-Estrogens

Dietary fiber influences sex hormone levels. It can diminish the intestinal re-uptake of estrogens by binding them up, causing more excretion in the feces. One outcome is that vegetarians, whose diets are generally high in fiber and low in fat, have significantly higher fecal bulk weights, and higher removal of estrogens.

Also very important—dietary fiber carries material called phytoestrogens, and these have antiestrogenic activity. Other dietary sources of antiestrogenic plant compounds come in the form of lignans. Lignans, if you recall, are structural components in plants that have potent beneficial biological activities.

The amount of lignans passed into the urine directly correlates with consumption of fruits, berries, legumes, grain fibers, and vegetable fibers. Strict vegetarians have elevated levels of urinary lignans and of plant estrogens compared to meat eaters. Lignans will bind weakly to estrogen receptors, tying them up and physically blocking estrogen's normal activity. Think of a key and a lock. The lignans act like rusty keys—not able to open the lock effectively, but blocking the real key, estrogen, from opening it. Indeed, studies have shown that women can significantly lower circulating levels of estrogen by changing to a low-fat/high-fiber diet

In addition, lignans and isoflavonoids have been proven to stimulate production of protein called the sex hormone binding globulin (SHGB). Extra SHGB binds up free estrogen, delaying its action and starving estrogen-dependent breast cancer cells.

Estrogen-lowering foods include: legumes, whole grains, berries, broccoli, and brussels sprouts.

Soy Protein

Soy proteins have shown exciting beneficial effects for both men and women. Soy protein is at the forefront of warding off breast cancer. A study in Singapore confirmed that a mere morsel of soy (55 mg/day) crushed breast cancer rates by 50 percent. Soy protein has also been shown to reduce lung cancer in China and prostate cancer in Japan. The Japanese consume soy daily in the form of tofu, soy milk, and fermented soy products such as miso.

All soy foods contain isoflavones, and research has zeroed in on a particular soy isoflavone called genistein. Impressively, genistein intercepts and stifles the growth of a wide variety of cancer cells, and hinders a number of proteins and enzymes which play key roles in cancer growth and regulation.

One of the main reasons soy protein may safeguard against breast cancer is its ability to delay the menstrual cycle by one to five days. It well known that Asian women have longer menstrual cycles than Western women. Asian women also have much easier transitions into menopause, and this explains why there is no cognate in the Japanese language for hot flashes.

Vitamins

Exciting results in reducing breast cancer rates are also surfacing through research on retinoids. Substances that are related to vitamin A, retinoids seem to hinder the transformation of malignant cells. This may be due to heightened communication between cells, since retinoids can also reverse the stages of precancer cells and restore normal growth regulation, thereby suppressing cancer cell growth. Several retinoids taken together may provide enhanced protection.

Vitamin D is also important in reducing breast cancer, with increased intake of both calcium and vitamin D showing good results.

Vitamin E has shown promise too. It has been discovered that the ductal portions of the breast store vitamin E in adequate concentrations to provide protection from cancer. The longer that vitamin E is taken, the greater the stored concentrations of vitamin E.

Measures to Prevent Breast Cancer

- Low-fat diet with little intake of animal products
- Exercise, which promotes the beneficial C-2 pathway for estrogen.
- Soy products
- Beta carotene
- Omega-3 fats
- Selenium
- Aspirin every 3 days, never on an empty stomach (enteric-coated aspirin will lessen stomach irritation)
- Olive oil, high-fiber, and lignans diet (fiber reduces the re-uptake of estrogens and lessens the chance of breast cancer)

- Licorice root extract
- Cruciferous vegetables
- Vitamin A
- Vitamin D
- Vitamin E
- Green tea
- Fenretinide, a synthetic retinoid
- Tamoxifen (though it may increase risk of ovarian cancer)
- Red onions, which are anti-estrogenic and inhibit the growth of human breast cancer cells in culture

Radiation

Radiation, on the other hand, is an unequivocal cause of breast cancer. It is not the only cause, of course. Inherited genes, fat, estrogen, estrogen-mimicking chemicals, and viruses cause breast cancer also, alone or in combination with radiation.

Mammography itself is radiation: an X-ray picture of the breast to detect a potential tumor. Each woman must weigh for herself the risks and benefits of mammography. As with most carcinogens, there is a latency period or delay between the time of irradiation and the occurrence of breast cancer. This delay can vary up to decades for different people. Response to radiation is especially dramatic in children. Women who received X-rays of the breast area as children have shown increased rates of breast cancer as adults. The first increase is reflected in women younger than thirty-five, who have early onset breast cancer. But for this exposed group, flourishing breast cancer rates continue for another forty years or longer.

Breast cancer is much more likely to result from radiation exposures than are other cancers. In fact, it is two to three times more apt to occur from radiation than cancers in other tissues and organs. What makes the female breast so sensitive to the effects of radiation is not fully understood. But after observing humans exposed to radiation in Hiroshima and Nagasaki, compelling evidence suggests that there is no safe dose of radiation. Any exposure carries some risk.

One strategy for intercepting cancer and sparing some radiation injury to the breast is the use of sulfur amino acids.

Methionine and cysteine are amino acids that contain sulfur, and they limit some of radiation's toxic effects. Therefore it seems prudent for a woman who is about to undergo diagnostic X-ray tests to supplement her diet prior to exposure with radioprotective amino acids like cysteine (see notes on DNA repair in chapters 3, 5 and 7).

Alcohol

Be cautious with alcohol. Studies of premenopausal women indicate that estrogen levels rise even with moderate consumption of alcohol. Women who drink heavily face a 40 to 100 percent chance of getting breast cancer. Alcohol has a bruising effect on melatonin, a naturally occurring hormone that acts as an antioxidant and combats cancer. Because alcohol reduces melatonin production, it inhibits the body's natural protection against cancer.

BENEFITS OF MELATONIN

decreases cancer cell growth

more potent antioxidant than vitamin E

increases the brain's major antioxidant enzyme

antiestrogenic

increases survival in cancer patients

Cervical Cancer

Cervical cancer is the second most common cancer in women. The cervix is considered to be the lower third of the uterus. In many countries cervical cancer is declining, due to widespread use of screening methods like the Pap smear.

Risk Factors for Cervical Cancer

A number of factors increase the risk of getting this cancer:

- Virus infection known as HPV (human papilloma virus)
- High number of sexual partners, which increases exposure to HPV
- Sexual activity at an early age, which increases contact with HPV
- Cigarette smoking, especially for long-term and high-intensity smokers
- Low dietary intake of carotenoids. Studies show that women with low intake of carotenoids, especially lycopene, have increased cancer rates

Anticancer Agents for the Cervix

- Folic acid (green vegetables, broccoli, bulgar, okra, orange juice, spinach, white beans, kidney beans, soybeans, wheat germ, asparagus, avocado, and brussels sprouts—especially critical for women who use oral contraceptives, which lower folic acid levels)
- Lycopene (tomatoes apparently prevent the precancerous signs of cervical cancer)
- Skim milk (low-fat and skim milk drinkers are less likely than whole milk drinkers to develop various cancers—cervical, oral, stomach, colon, lung, bladder, and breast)
- Vitamin C (especially protective against cervical cancer in smokers)
- Vitamin E
- Vitamin A analogues, such as retinoic acid which—according to one study—caused a regression in cancer when topically applied to the cervical area
- Vegetarian diets

Ovarian Cancer

Cancer of the ovary is very difficult to detect since there are no reliable screening methods. But data show that Asian women have a low incidence of ovarian cancer. While there may be genetic factors, the likelyhood, here again, is that Asian diets prevent cancer.

Risk Factors for Ovarian Cancer

- High intake of animal fat or red meat
- Coffee (decaffeinated coffee did not seem to increase risk)
- Lack of childbearing (the more ovulations in a woman's life, the greater her risk of ovarian cancer)
- Family history
- Early age of menstruation
- Fertility drugs (hormones used to stimulate ovulation are linked to increased risk of ovarian cancer

- Use of talc (which can be contaminated with asbestos, a known carcinogen)[1]
- Herbicides (one study linked herbicide exposure to ovarian cancer)
- High intake of dairy products (which may cause cancer through dairy fats or lactose sugar, especially in those with lactose intolerance)
- Tamoxifen (used to prevent breast cancer) has been shown to increase the rise of ovarian cancer
- Any high-dose radiation exposure

Ovarian Cancer Blockers

- Asian diet (a diet low in animal products and high in fresh fruits and vegetables is protective)
- High vegetable fiber intake which strongly reduces the chance of ovarian cancer. (every 10 grams, 0.35 ounces, of vegetable fiber reflects a 37 percent decrease in cancer risk)
- Vegetarian diets (based on fresh fruits and vegetables)
- Oral contraceptives (when used for one year, the pill reduces the risk of ovarian cancer by 10 percent; when used for five to ten, the risk falls to 50 percent)
- Low animal fat diets
- Breastfeeding (the longer the breastfeeding period, the more protection is gained)
- Pregnancy (one pregnancy may reduce incidence rates by as much as 50 percent)

Uterine Cancer

Uterine, or endometrial, cancer is the most common female cancer in

RISK FACTORS FOR UTERINE CANCER

obesity—the risk of endometrial cancer is elevated in women who are significantly overweight

high dietary fat—from animal products

high dietary protein—from animal products

excess estrogen—synthetic estrogen replacement therapy is linked to increased uterine cancer

late menopause—women who experience late menopause have more menstrual cycles, and therefore elevated risks

(vegetarian diets with a high daily intake of complex carbohydrates, including green vegetables and fruit, are protective against uterine cancer)

[1] Talc use in the groin area has been shown to migrate internally, eventually reaching the ovaries.

the United States. The endometrium is the mucous membrane comprising the inner wall of the uterus. Endometrial cancer arises on the inner layer of the uterine wall.

Chapter Recap

- Breast cancer is showing an alarming increase in countries all over the world.

- Soy products, cruciferous vegetables, vitamins, minerals, and omega-3 fats are linked to preventing breast cancer.

- As a general rule avoid consuming animal products in order to protect against cancers of the breast, ovary, cervix, and uterus.

- Breast cancer, and other female cancers, can be largely prevented by reducing or eliminating risk factors, and by consuming an anticancer diet (as outlined in the meal plan earlier in chapter 6).

Cancer Busting for Mothers & Children

A series of fascinating studies have reflected the beneficial effects of the cancer-busting regimen for children, pregnant mothers, and even fathers-to-be.

Protecting Your Child

Young children are at increased risk from toxic substances due to a number of factors. Very young children do not have fully developed protective systems. For example, humans have a specialized blood vessel system in the brain called the blood brain barrier (BBB). In young children the BBB is not yet fully operational. So many chemicals that are easily excluded by the adult brain will readily pass into the brain of an infant or a young child.

The destiny of nations depends on the manner wherein they take their food.

—Anthelme Brillat-Savarin, 1755–1826

Also, young children will put nonfood items in their mouths, so they are more exposed than adults to environmental agents such as dust and lead. You can actually increase your children's intelligence if you can prevent their exposure to lead. Lead's health consequences for children are serious because by the time toxic symptoms are discovered, irreversible damage to the nervous system has already occurred. A permanently dulled intelligence is often the unfortunate result of lead toxicity. The up side is that lead toxicity is completely preventable.

Ways to Reduce Lead Exposure
- Use lead-free bottled water.
- Check tap water for lead. Use an EPA-certified lab to test your drinking water. If tap water has detectable lead, install a filtration system, especially for the water used in food preparation.
- Do not use ceramic dishes. Ceramic, pottery, or earthenware dishes have varying levels of lead. Do not feed children from these unless they are lead-free.
- Check soil lead levels. Remove contaminated soils from your child's play area. Soil immediately near outside walls may have been contaminated from paint renovations.

- Test paint, dishes, and other substances with a lead kit (see appendixes D and F).
- Keep children away from colored newsprint. Colored newsprint contains lead compounds and should not be burned in fireplaces.
- Use a HEPA vacuum cleaner. High-Efficiency Particulate Air-filtered vacuums remove small dust particles that conventional vacuums do not.
- Limit a child's exposure to cosmetics and dark hair dyes that contain lead.
- Limit the use of canned foods (especially imported) since they may have high levels of lead.
- Avoid hobbies that use lead: furniture refinishing, stained glass windows, indoor firing ranges (primer in bullets contains lead), pool-cue chalk (contains lead), and lead-glazed pottery.
- Use lead-free calcium supplements (see appendix D).

A sensible amount of dietary calcium can help battle lead since calcium competes with lead for absorption. If children are calcium-deficient they will be sopping up more lead. Be cautious when selecting calcium supplements since some bone meals may also contain lead.

Infants and children are especially sensitive to toxic substances because children absorb more than adults, the substances exert more damage to them, toxic substances are not removed from their systems as quickly as adults, and a child's lifestyle leads to greater exposure.

Women's Preparations

During pregnancy there is an increased requirement for the essential nutrient folic acid. If pregnant women have folic acid deficiencies, they're at risk of having babies with nervous system defects. The richest and most common sources of folic acid are dark green leafy vegetables.

Years before conception women should:

- Eat organic foods
- Limit smoking (which increases lead and cadmium in the infant)

- Limit alcohol and the use of drugs
- Avoid chemical exposures
- Take time-release vitamin C and antioxidant supplements such as vitamin E and beta carotene (see Chapter 7)
- Follow the cancer-busting regimen

Because of widespread mercury and environmental chemical contamination (PCBs), limit consumption of meat, fish, and poultry. Try to eat organic foods if possible, and get plenty of calcium-rich foods to counter the absorption of lead.

After the birth of a baby, the diet of both infant and mother remains vitally important. The mother should restrict her own intake of dairy before and after birth, until she stops breastfeeding. Once the infant is eating solid food, serve organic baby food for at least two years. Organic baby foods can be found at most health food stores. Do not feed an infant dairy products since this can lead to milk intolerance and diabetes.

Nature Does It Better

Over a hundred years ago Oliver Wendell Holmes said, "A pair of substantial mammary glands has the advantage over the two hemispheres of the most learned professor's brain in the art of compounding a nutritious fluid for infants."

To this day that statement remains true. Breastfeeding confers benefits no infant formula can ever hope to provide. Mother's milk transfers critical antibodies and essential fatty acids that are necessary for the growth of the newborn brain. Many commercial infant formulas lack essential fatty acids. Yet companies have marketed infant formulas and created a market that need not even exist (unless the mother or baby is too ill to nurse).

Benefits of Breast Feeding

- Fewer allergies result from breast milk than from any other infant food
- Transfer of antibodies to the infant
- Essential fats for brain growth

- Essential minerals (breast milk is nutritionally superior to any infant formula)
- Vitamins
- Trace minerals
- Promotes mother to child bonding
- Fresh and safe from bacterial contamination, unlike infant formulas
- Less expensive than infant formulas
- Breastfed infants less likely to be overfed
- More convenient than infant formulas

Men's Preparations

Conventional medical wisdom often overlooks the contribution of the male in conception. However, researchers have recently documented that vitamin C levels of seminal fluid are eight times higher than the levels of vitamin C circulating in blood. It seems that concentrated vitamin C wards off damage to the sperm. The study had men vary their daily intake of vitamin C while it monitored their sperm. This research found that men who received the lowest amounts of vitamin C each day pulverized their DNA, causing twice the amount of oxidative damage to DNA in their sperm as the men who received higher amounts. This should be a warning for male smokers who have greatly depleted levels of vitamin C. It has become apparent that a man's exposure to chemicals can influence his ability to parent a child, and that exposure can also determine the future health of his children. So real men eat organic vegetables; the fact is, men who eat organic vegetables have higher sperm counts than men who consume commercial produce.

Sperm have a three-month cycle. Therefore 90 days before conception is a critical period for men to preserve the integrity of the DNA in their sperm. This can be accomplished by limiting exposure to damaging chemicals and also by increasing their intake of antioxidants. Men exposed to paint solvents are at risk of fathering children with central nervous system defects.

Ninety Days Before Conception
Men should also prepare themselves for their partners' pregnancies:

- Limit smoking (which causes an oxidative threat to sperm)
- Limit alcohol and the use of drugs
- Avoid chemical exposures to paints, solvents, and other industrial and household chemicals
- Take time-release vitamin C and other antioxidant supplements such as vitamin E and beta carotene
- Follow the cancer-busting regimen

Chapter Recap

- Mothers and fathers alike should prepare themselves for conception by eating an anticancer diet.
- By taking some simple precautions your children can enjoy better health.
- Special care should be taken to keep the pregnant mother and the newborn child away from sources of lead.
- For the mother who has been eating the right diet, breast milk is the best possible nutritional source for her child.

The Cancer-Conquering Male: Defeating Prostate Cancer and Other Male Cancers

It is often joked that sex will be the next thing discovered to cause cancer. In fact research shows that men who have multiple partners and a greater frequency of sex may be boosting their chances of getting prostate cancer. One out of every six American men now contract this cancer. To prevent prostate cancer and still have a healthy sex life, the most sensible change a man can make is to eat more cancer-stifling foods!

> We owe it to ourselves to understand the disease and how to prevent it. It should be a top priority. Cancer isn't something that just happens to other people, it can happen to anyone.
>
> —Scott Hamilton, Olympic skater, 1997 (upon his diagnosis of testicular cancer)

Prostate Cancer

Global incidence of prostate cancer varies greatly. Low rates of prostate cancer occur in the Far East; moderate rates in south and western Europe; while very high rates exist in northern Europe and the United States. Cancer of the prostate is now the most common cancer among American men.

For unknown reasons, blacks in the U.S. manifest the highest rates in the world for prostate cancer. Exposure to sunlight is the biggest source of vitamin D, and since men with darker pigmented skin absorb less sun, it stands to reason that their levels of vitamin D would be lower. When researchers compared levels of vitamin D in black men in sun-drenched Zaire with black men who had moved to northern Europe, the men who moved to northern Europe showed much lower levels of vitamin D, and their incidence of prostate cancer was higher.

Scandinavian countries suffer an extremely high death rate from prostate cancer, while Japan's rate is low. The U.S. lies somewhere in between. Interestingly, Japanese men who immigrate to the U.S. have an incidence rate close to that of men born in the U.S. Japanese men living in Hawaii show a rate of prostate cancer that is lower than the continental U.S. rate. But it is still higher than for men in Japan.

The clear message from migration studies is that most prostate cancer is due to diet and to environmental factors, not genetics.

In the decade from 1980 to 1990, prostate cancer increased by about 50 percent. Every year nearly 200,000 new cases are diagnosed in the U.S. The prime increase is in men over age fifty, and it is the leading cause of death in men 75 years old and older.

Clearly, disease of the prostate gland is a major health issue for men. However, surgical removal of the prostate has a number of significant risks.

Since many of the nerves required for bladder control and erection are contained within the prostate gland, surgery to remove the prostate may also remove some of these nerves, rendering a man impotent or unable to control his bladder. Obviously, men should enthusiastically eat to beat prostate cancer.

The Prostate Gland

The prostate functions as a male accessory sex organ that contributes a milky substance to the semen. This secretion has an alkaline pH that serves to neutralize the seminal fluid, which is acidic. This enhances mobility of the sperm cells.

The prostate gland surrounds the beginning of the urethra, just below the bladder. The urethra is the tube leading from the bladder to the outside of the body. Enclosed by a capsule of connective tissue, the prostate consists of branched tubular glands and ducts that open into the urethra.

In Western men the walnut-sized prostate gland continues to grow throughout life. In male children the prostate is relatively small. It first begins to grow in early adolescence, and grows slowly from then on. As a rule it does not grow noticeably large until men reach their mid-forties. Thereafter, it may grow so big that it obstructs the flow of urine and impinges on the bladder wall. This results in frequent urination, especially at night. The size of the prostate gland of a sixty-five-year-old man is two to three times larger than that of a twenty-year-old. Beginning in the fifth decade of life, there is a progressive increase in prostate size. At the age of eighty, almost 80 percent of men have prostate enlargement.

The prostate has a strong tendency to undergo abnormal growth. But in modern times what is considered normal growth? What triggers the prostate gland to evolve from a lazy tumor into a life-threatening disease?

One leading clue is that cancer of the prostate is recognized in two forms. One is a small, dormant, localized cancer. The other is an active, energetic, particularly invasive cancer. Whether these are two different paths the disease takes or two different stages is uncertain, since the dormant and aggressive forms are indistinguishable under a microscope, except for size.

The three important questions are these: What is responsible for the continuous growth of the prostate gland throughout life? What occurs to change this into a life-threatening disease? Is the progression toward prostate cancer inevitable?

It is now accepted that a large number of men with prostate cancer have long, stable periods without tumor growth. This is the period when cancer-crushing agents in the diet can be the most effective in halting or arresting the inevitable tumor growth. The various growth rates of the tumor are the most confusing aspect of the disease. Many men develop symptoms of prostate cancer, but they end up dying of other causes before the prostate tumor spreads to other tissues.

Sex Hormones

As in breast cancer in women, hormones also play a central role in prostate cancer. As a male accessory sex organ, the prostate gland is extremely sensitive to the effects of male hormones.

The testes produce 90 percent of the circulating male hormones (androgens). Some data suggest that men with elevated testosterone levels have a higher risk of prostate cancer. Higher testosterone levels have also been associated with Western (but not vegetarian) diets. In that light, it is interesting to note that men in Japan and Taiwan have some of the lowest rates of prostate cancer in the world.

In any case, male hormones regulate the growth, differentiation, and even the shape of the prostate. Throughout a man's life his hormones change, and so does the prostate gland.

An intact hormone supply seems to be a requirement for development of prostate cancer. Prostate cancer simply does not occur in eunuchs, men castrated at an early age, and men with low levels of testosterone. Prostate cancer also shows a close correlation with age, regardless of which global population is examined.

It is now believed that the metabolic products of testosterone cause an enlarged prostate and cancer. Within the prostate gland, the hormone testosterone is rapidly and irreversibly converted by an enzyme to a more potent product called DHT.

Amazingly, green tea, essential fatty acids, and berries help to keep the enzyme in check that converts testosterone into DHT. Another interesting note: German studies show that the natural compound (saw palmetto extract) is more effective and has less side effects, than the prescription drug commonly used to treat enlarged prostate glands.

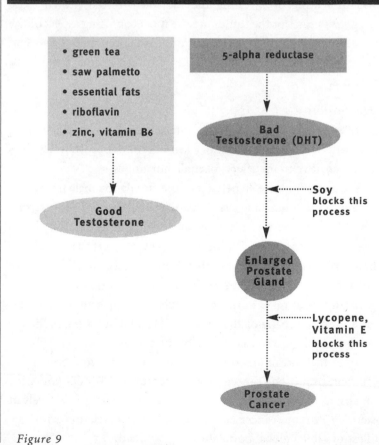

METABOLISM OF TESTOSTERONE WITHIN THE PROSTATE GLAND

- green tea
- saw palmetto
- essential fats
- riboflavin
- zinc, vitamin B6

5-alpha reductase

Bad Testosterone (DHT)

Good Testosterone

Soy blocks this process

Enlarged Prostate Gland

Lycopene, Vitamin E blocks this process

Prostate Cancer

Figure 9

When men are first diagnosed with prostate cancer, 75 percent have tumors that respond at least partially to withdrawal of male hormones like testosterone. Tragically, almost all prostate cancer sufferers will also eventually develop hormone-independent tumors. Clinicians do not know how to treat these hormone-independent cancers.

Prevention Meal Plan

The following diet is particularly good in preventing prostate cancer:
- Soybean products (soya and soy products, soy milk, tofu)
- ODC inhibitors (licorice, carrots, wheat, garlic, onions, asparagus, cucumbers, tomatoes, strawberries, citrus)— ornithine decarboxylase is an enzyme
- Cruciferous vegetables (radishes, potatoes, spices like turmeric, high levels of calcium)
- Protease inhibitors (seeds, nuts, legumes, beans, squash zucchini, rice, barley, rye, oats, cucumber seeds, potatoes)
- Fruits (strawberries, raspberries)
- Alpha-5-reductase enzyme inhibitor (saw palmetto berry extract, berries, green tea, riboflavin, essential fats)
- Vitamins and minerals (vitamins C, E, beta carotene, selenium, and particularly vitamin D)
- Retinoids (tomatoes and watermelon—lycopene[1]—carrots)
- Miscellaneous—green tea, licorice, pumpkin seeds, zinc[2]

Be sure to avoid:
- Diets high in saturated fats
- Safflower oil, corn oil, sunflower oil, and cottonseed oil
- Red meat and organ meats
- Anabolic steroids
- Excessive seafood and shellfish
- Dairy products

---

[1] A recent study showed reduced prostate cancer in men who frequently consumed baked tomato products. Lycopene is a retinoid found in tomatoes and watermelon that does not stay in the body long. A daily infusion of baked tomato products or watermelon is recommended.

[2] Zinc is concentrated in the prostate gland more than any other organ. The toxic metal cadmium competes for absorption with zinc. Therefore, plenty of zinc in the diet not only hinders the uptake of cadmium but also may impede its toxicity.

Diet and Related Factors

Long ago tomatoes were believed to be deadly aphrodisiacs. Now tomatoes have a lofty status; they are more important to the health of the prostate gland than anyone previously imagined. Harvard researchers found that men who get at least ten servings of tomato-based foods per week are 45 percent less likely to develop prostate cancer.

Lycopene is a retinoid found in abundance in tomato products and watermelon. Lycopene is the most abundant carotenoid stored in the prostate gland, and it is more potent than beta carotene in protecting against prostate cancer. But lycopene is not stored for very long, which means that a daily dose of lycopene-rich food is in every man's best interest. Lycopene is absorbed better when tomatoes are cooked with olive oil or baked. If you cannot include tomato-based foods in your diet, then take lycopene supplements (see appendix F). Also, limit synthetic fat intake, since it reduces beta carotene and the amount of lycopene in the body.

Obesity
Nine out of ten studies have shown increasing risk for prostate cancer with increasing degrees of obesity. Most studies found that men who eat oversized portions of meat or dairy products are 30 to 50 percent more apt to get prostate cancer. The evidence is quite consistent that meat, dairy products, animal fat, and total fat are associated with increased prostate cancer risk.

Men who eat red meat five or more times per week face a 2.5 times greater risk of developing prostate cancer than men who eat meat once a week or less. On the other hand, a prostate-cancer reducing wallop has been linked in Japan with soy protein and soy products.

Risk Factors for Prostate Cancer
A number of studies have shown correlations between lifestyle, experience and family history. While virtually no one can escape all of these factors, if a number of them are true of you, you should recognize you are a higher risk than the rest of the population.

- Age (many men over 40 begin to experience prostate difficulties)
- Family history (men whose fathers or brothers have prostate cancer are twice as likely to suffer the same condition)
- Vitamin D deficiency
- Ethnic background (Americans of African descent have highest rates)
- Sexually transmitted diseases, such as genital warts
- Sexual relations with multiple partners
- Obesity (overweight men have a 2.5 times greater chance for fatal prostate cancer than men closer to ideal body weight)
- Western diet (animal fat from red meat—not vegetable fat—seems to create the main danger)
- Cadmium exposure (which, as mentioned earlier, antagonizes zinc, an essential trace element)
- Radiation (which increases the risk of cancer)
- Anabolic steroid use (higher testosterone and DHEA levels increase likelihood of cancer)
- Farm environment (risk for farmers may be related to pesticide exposure)
- Low vegetable intake (men who rarely eat green and yellow vegetables have twice the chance of getting prostate cancer)
- Vasectomy (prostate cancer seems to be greater in men who had a vasectomy performed over twenty years ago)
- Industrial chemicals, such as those used by rubber companies
- Dairy products (a growth factor in milk—elevated in dairy cows treated with growth hormones—was linked to prostate cancer by a Harvard study)

ANTICANCER AGENTS FOR THE PROSTATE

carrots—retinoids

tomatoes—lycopene, a retinoid, is found in baked tomato products, red grapefruit, and watermelon

yellow and green vegetables—asparagus, carrots, lettuce, parsley, leeks, green peppers, chives, pumpkin, and spinach

saw palmetto berries—with essential fats, these help block conversion of testosterone to more potent DHT

vitamin D

soy products, which contain protective isoflavones

ODC inhibitors—licorice root extract

protease inhibitors

low-fat diet

strawberries and berries

pumpkin seeds

selenium

green tea—blocks formation of DHT and an enzyme called urokinase, which is critical for cancer growth

exercise

Vitamins

Recent studies suggest that beta carotene supplements are not a key factor in combating the risk of prostate cancer. Yet the matter is not that simple, since carrots containing beta carotene do reduce the risk. While carrots protect, no consistent patterns were shown for green vegetables. Bottom line: Get your beta carotene from food, not from supplements!

Widely publicized studies show that vitamin E also acts as a bodyguard against prostate cancer. And men with high levels of circulating vitamin D have a lower rate of prostate cancer.

The critical message: There is a tremendous opportunity for men to forestall the progression of prostate cancer by including more cancer-crushing agents in their diets.

Testicular Cancer

Testicular cancer has increased worldwide in the last thirty years. Testicular cancer is a young man's cancer, most commonly found in fifteen- to thirty-five-year-olds. Unfortunately, no one really knows what factors lead to development of testicular cancer.

RISK FACTORS FOR TESTICULAR CANCER

tight-fitting underwear

men born to women given estrogen

inadequate exercise

undescended testes at birth

diet high in saturated fat

testicular trauma

estrogen-mimicking pollutants like PCBs

Some clues come from Danish men, who face an unusually high risk when compared with their Scandinavian neighbors. During World War II, Denmark was isolated from the outside world by German occupation, so high-fat animal products were in short supply. Men who were born during this period of isolation showed a decreased risk of testicular cancer, compared with men born either before or after the war. It has been suggested that the war diet, one low in animal products, was responsible for less testicular cancer. In the present day, however, Denmark tops the globe, reflecting the highest incidence rate of testicular cancer in the world.

The U.S. is also experiencing a dramatic increase in testicular cancer, suggesting that environmental factors are at play. One study conducted in Los Angeles found that men whose mothers had been given estrogen during pregnancy were eight times more likely to have testicular cancer than men whose mothers had not been given estrogen. This study and others have focused on maternal exposures of both estrogen-mimicking chemicals and pollutants as environmental factors in testicular cancer. Chemicals such as PCBs and organochlorine compounds are also linked to decreased sperm counts.

PREVENTION GENERAL MEAL PLAN

low saturated-fat diet— little red meat

Japanese or Oriental diet

vitamins and minerals —C, E, selenium

follow the diet to prevent prostate cancer

Another risk factor in testicular cancer is undescended testes (cryptochidism) at birth. The testes normally descend into the external scrotum during the seventh month of pregnancy. When the testes have not descended before birth, men have an increased cancer risk. Studies in England have shown that from the 1950's to the mid-1980's, the rate of undescended testes increased by 65 to 100 percent.

Chapter Recap

- Cancer of the prostate gland is on the rampage. It is now the most common cancer of American men.
- Current treatment for prostate cancer has undesirable side effects.
- A male's dietary choices are critical in preventing prostate and testicular cancer.
- High-fat animal products are a consistent risk factor for prostate and testicular cancer.
- The most practical, sensible changes a man can make concern the intake of cancer-stifling foods such as soy, green tea, and lycopene.

Fortify Your Lifestyle:
What to Eat if You Smoke or Drink Alcohol

Historians have noted that cancer often rises in proportion to the progress of civilization. The more affluent the society, the greater the chance of cancer. This is certainly true of Americans, who indulge in lifestyles that include tobacco and alcohol. Of course humans vary in their individual response to any kind of chemical agents. And a host of confounding factors may influence your chemical responses, including your age, gender, nutritional status, and state of health.

Unless we change direction we are likely to end up where we are headed.

—Ancient Chinese Proverb

The last ten years have brought unprecedented breakthroughs in our understanding of how food can affect chemical behavior and health. Yet you might not be aware that food choices can fortify against the ill effects of tobacco and alcohol, and even promote the birth of healthier children.

High-Risk Habits

We have all heard it before: Tobacco smoking is known to cause cancer. The message is emblazoned on the sides of cigarette packages. Yet the vast majority of smokers don't realize that their diet can help protect against the cancer threat.

Japan—a country with one of the highest per capita rates of cigarette consumption in the world—has one of the world's lowest lung cancer rates. The Japanese smoke like chimneys, yet if you live in Japan you will probably eat watercress, drink green tea, and not get lung cancer if you smoke. This bit of information leads one to conclude that powerful factors other than cigarettes are involved in the development of lung cancer.

If you must smoke, your approach to nutrition can save your life. If you have a significant other who smokes, make sure that person uses filtered, low-tar, light or blond tobacco, and adds cancer-slashing agents to the daily diet.

Cancer-Slashing Agents to Combat Tobacco Smoke

- Vitamins A, C, and E. Time-release vitamin C is highly recommended
- Beta carotene
- B vitamins, especially vitamin B12
- Folic acid
- Zinc
- Cruciferous vegetables (fresh watercress)
- Citrus fruit oils
- Red wine
- Green tea
- Ellagic acid (berries)
- Lycopene (low levels of lycopene can triple the lung cancer risk)
- Light, low-tar tobacco (low-tar, filtered cigarettes have dramatically less risk of lung cancer than non-filtered, high-tar cigarettes)

TOBACCO-RELATED ILLNESSES

stomach and intestinal ulcers

cancer of the mouth, throat, kidney, bladder, pancreas, and cervix

low birth weight in infants from mothers who smoke

infertility in men, decreased motility of sperm

emotional instability, increased cataracts, reduced peripheral vision and visual acuity, osteoporosis in women

slow healing of wounds and aortic aneurysm

Despite costly efforts by society to eliminate smoking, people continue to smoke. It is difficult to find a disease that is not linked in some way to tobacco use. Yet regrettably people will continue to smoke. Your dietary choices, however, can be important factors in reducing the possibility of lung cancer.

The ill health effects of smoking are endless: atherosclerosis, coronary heart disease, cerebrovascular disease, lung cancer, emphysema, and chronic obstructive lung disease, among others.

Since the number of males who smoke in Japan is twice the number in the United States, studies are puzzling that show deaths from lung cancer in Japanese males to be significantly lower than for American men. In both Japan and China, 60 to 70 percent of the men smoke. Yet in both countries the incidence of coronary heart disease is also very low.

Once again it becomes clear that diet can either protect you or it can make you more susceptible to the ill effects of tobacco use. For example, in China almost 90 percent of the people follow the protective dietary customs of drinking green tea and eating an enormous amount of cabbage. Green tea can protect from tobacco smoke toxicity, and cabbage is high in vitamins C and E.

Tobacco smoke is a complex mixture containing over 4,000 identified components. When tobacco burns it causes unstable, highly reactive compounds called free radicals to form. Free radicals are molecules that have an imbalance in their electrons that compels them to be reactionary, so they race wildly around in your cells searching for more electrons. By tearing electrons away from otherwise stable molecules they incite a cellular riot, starting a cascade of toxic insults that in time can cripple the cell. These highly toxic free radicals degrade fats (lipid peroxidation) and proteins, disable critical enzymes, mangle DNA, and disrupt the cell to the point where it can burst like a balloon.

Cigarette smoke has two phases, a tar phase and a gas phase, and both phases create free radicals that cause tissue injury in smokers. The particulate or tar portion of smoke contains free radicals that are relatively stable. More free radicals are contained in the gas phase. The free radical load from cigarette smoking appears to be counteracted by both vitamins C and E. In fact, it is believed that vitamins C and E are primary in preventing free-radical-mediated tissue damage and cancer.

Studies show that tobacco smoke damages the fat, or low-density lipoproteins (LDL) circulating in the blood. LDLs do not attach to the blood vessel wall in their normal form. They must first be damaged by free radicals, then ingested by white blood cells to become foam cells. Foam cells give rise to yellow fatty streaks, which are a hallmark of heart disease. Evidence suggests that the LDL membranes do not undergo damage until all of the available antioxidants, such as vitamin E and beta carotene, have been used up. Since smokers are shown to have reduced blood levels of these antioxidants, it appears that cigarette smoke may strip the LDL of any antioxidant capacity.

Several nutrients like carotenoids from fruits and vegetables show a protective role in smokers. In the lungs of heavy cigarette smokers, retinoids like beta carotene can reverse cells that are disturbed and almost cancerous, turning them back into normal cells.

Vitamin E has been shown to reduce damage done by free radicals from cigarette smoke. Zinc may have similar protective features. Tobacco use may affect zinc levels since tobacco smoke contains cadmium, which competes with zinc for uptake from the intestine.

Vitamin E and zinc may also be protective in heart and vascular diseases. The essential mineral zinc is a component of membranes, necessary for their structure and function. A deficiency of dietary zinc has been shown to decrease plasma concentrations of vitamin E, suggesting that zinc deficiency may increase your nutritional requirements for vitamin E. High zinc foods include pumpkin seeds, peanuts, squash seeds, legumes, turkey (dark meat), oysters and shellfish (though seafood should be eaten sparingly).

It is now well documented that snacking on vegetables can protect you from lung cancer caused by smoking. The precise nature of the substances in vegetables that may be responsive is not known. Crucifers like broccoli and cauliflower have a stronger association with reducing risk of lung cancer than does beta carotene.

Alcohol and Drug Use

Excessive alcohol use (more than five drinks per day) has been associated with cancer of the mouth, esophagus, and liver. Toxic compounds such as acetaldehyde are created when alcohol is processed by the liver. However, it seems that vitamin C protects from some of the toxicity associated with acetaldehyde.

There is ample data to show that alcoholic beverages can cause cancer. Keep in mind that many alcoholic beverages are complex mixtures that contain potent toxic chemicals other than alcohol. Nitrates contained in

---

COUNTERACTING ALCOHOL

If you drink alcohol, make sure you get adequate amounts of:

selenium

vitamin A—alcohol decreases vitamin A storage and increases the toxicity of vitamin A

vitamin C—very important

vitamin E

thiamin

choline

vitamins B6 and B12

green vegetables

glutathione

folic acid

methionine

zinc

biotin

riboflavin

melatonin—alcohol inhibits the release of melatonin, an antioxidant that is linked with decreasing toxicity and decreasing cancer

niacin

beer and scotch are known to be converted into potent carcinogens. If you drink, choose red wine.

There is no doubt that alcohol exerts its toxicity by the combined effects of malnutrition and production of the highly toxic acetaldehyde. However consumption of green vegetables seems to be a modifying factor in reducing cancer risk from alcohol. Alcohol profoundly affects the way folic acid is treated by the body. In fact a deficiency of folic acid has been associated with excessive alcohol consumption for many years. Vitamin E, thiamin, and glutathione also show up as nutritional deficiencies. Alcoholics with thiamin deficits frequently have heart problems. Nutritional deficiencies may be at the bottom of alcohol toxicity. Therefore, if a person regularly drinks alcohol, he or she needs heightened nutritional awareness. (See chapter 7 on vitamins.)

People who regularly abuse alcohol have low levels of vitamin A in their livers. But this is not totally due to poor uptake. Alcohol stimulates the activity of the liver, which in turn causes vitamin A to be broken down at a higher rate in the liver. Finally the presence of alcohol causes increased movement of vitamin A from the liver to other tissues.

Alcohol also causes an accelerated breakdown of vitamin E. Since vitamin E and glutathione are required for the liver's normal detoxification processes, these nutritional deficiencies can directly lead to toxic consequences. Cell membranes are then destroyed, with one result being alcoholic liver disease.

In addition, alcohol can interfere with vitamin D function. Since vitamin D is crucial to maintaining calcium and bone formation, a lifetime of alcohol consumption will disrupt calcium actions in the body and can lead to osteoporosis.

Zinc deficiency is often observed in heavy drinkers. This deficiency leads to enhanced activation of carcinogens like nitrosamines in the throat surface. In fact, low blood levels of zinc and vitamin A are associated with throat cancer. Concurrently, high intakes of zinc and vitamin A are associated with less throat cancer.

Light to moderate drinking of alcohol also slows down the burning of fats, leading to increased fat storage (probably the reason why people become overweight when they regularly drink even moderate amounts of alcohol). If moderate to light drinkers will reduce their fat intake, this can help to avoid the potential weight gain due to ethanol. Bottom line: If you drink, try to consume only low-fat foods.

Regular alcohol use can increase the toxicity of over-the-counter and prescription drugs, as well as environmental chemicals. It is wise to follow the old adage that says, "Make not thy stomach an apothecary's shop." Lower your intake of prescription and over-the-counter drugs. Physicians are likely to overprescribe drugs due to increasing malpractice lawsuits; if they fail to prescribe a preferred drug and you develop complications, there are grounds for a malpractice suit. But it is your choice to fill the prescription or not. Of course if you have a life-threatening illness (like asthma, for example) you have no choice but to take medication.

But use your common sense in avoiding the overprescribed, frivolous drugs. For instance antidiarrhea drugs do stop the symptoms of diarrhea, but they do nothing for the real cause, which is usually food-borne bacteria. In the long run it is healthier to allow diarrhea to run its course, clearing your system of the disease-producing bacteria, rather than using a drug to interrupt the body's normal defenses.

It is wise to be aware and be careful. Even over-the-counter drugs are capable of causing severe maladies. For instance, the common drug acetaminophen reduces glutathione levels in the liver, but glutathione is needed for normal liver detoxification. Many drugs are processed by the body in exactly the same way that environmental pollutants are, and they therefore become an additional burden on the body's clearance systems.

Chapter Recap

- Dietary choices can diminish the toxicity of high-risk habits like tobacco smoking, alcohol, and drugs.

Beating Other Important Cancers

Many other types of cancer afflict people in the United States. The cancers in this chapter are listed in order of decreasing incidence, from the most prevalent to the least.

Lung Cancer

Lung cancer remains a perennial killer; in fact it continues to be a leading cause of cancer death in most countries. The known causes of lung cancer range from radon and other pollutants, to active and passive smoking. In recent decades, dietary components that have shown a consistent pattern of reducing lung cancer are fresh fruits and vegetables.

We've poured in many billions of dollars in an effort to find improved cancer treatments, we've given it our very best scientific talent, and it just hasn't worked. It's time to recognize it hasn't worked. It's time to get serious about prevention.

—Dr. John C. Bailar III, Chair, Department of Health Studies, University of Chicago

Lung Cancer Risk Factors

- Tobacco (filtered cigarettes have less risk compared with nonfiltered; low-tar—blonde—tobacco has one-fourth the risk of high tar)
- Passive smoke (lung cancer risk is elevated by passive inhalation of tobacco smoke)
- Exposure to arsenic, asbestos, and chromium (usually from occupations)
- Radon and polycyclic hydrocarbons
- Silica
- High saturated fat intake (high levels of certain fats and cholesterol increase risk of lung cancer)
- Red meat or high-protein diets (women who consume a lot of red meat are twice as likely to get lung cancer)
- Lycopene (very low levels of lycopene can triple the lung cancer risk)
- Obesity
- Radiation

ANTICANCER AGENTS FOR LUNG CANCER

fresh fruits and vegetables— cantaloupe, oranges, spinach, kale, carrots, broccoli, onions, pumpkin, sweet potatoes, beans, dark green and yellow leafy vegetables, yellow-orange vegetables, citrus fruit

beta carotene

lycopene

vitamins A, C, E

green tea

The Japanese drink green tea daily and have the lowest rates of lung cancer in the world. Green tea can block cancer-causing substances in tobacco and prevent lung cancers in mice.

Large Intestine Cancer

The large intestine is a 4- to 5-foot length of tubing that maintains intimate contact with ingested food. So diet has a crucial influence on cancer within the intestines. Cancer of the large intestine is second only to lung cancer in terms of its death rate. While controversy exists among cancer studies of the colon, rectum, and large intestine, general agreement is emerging as to the risk factors.

ANTICANCER AGENTS FOR THE LARGE INTESTINE

high fruit and vegetable intake, major sources for vitamins C, E, beta carotene, folic acid, selenium, zinc

high-fiber diet

low animal-fat diet

high intake of vitamin E

green and black tea, known to inhibit the growth of bacteria (Clostridium botulinum) associated with intestinal cancer

calcium and vitamin D

exercise—reduced colon cancer by 50 percent in people who exercised by walking 1 hour a day

folic acid also reduces risk of colon cancer

Risk Factors

- Heterocyclic amines (potent DNA toxic agents are formed from charbroiling, frying, and high-temperature cooking)
- Bile acids (which are converted into more toxic secondary bile acids by intestinal bacteria, and high dietary fat increases bile secretion)
- Animal protein and fat (incidence of intestinal cancer increases in countries with high intakes of animal products, especially beef)
- High-fat diet (more tumor promoting compounds are formed with low-fiber/high-fat diets)
- Low-fiber diet
- High caloric intake (which increases the risk of large intestine cancer)
- Alcoholic beverages (some studies have shown excessive beer to increase the risk of rectal cancer)
- Cigarette smoke

Skin Cancer

The dark side of sunlight is skin cancer. Skin cancer is increasing, largely as a result of desires for a glowing tan. While a tan exudes the appearance of health, the warmth of the sun is silently ravaging your skin. No one seems to argue that overexposure to the sun will cause skin cancer.

In the 18th century the fashion-conscious covered their faces with white powders, since at that time the pale look was in vogue. In modern times a bronzed look has become the aesthetic. The production of melanin, a dark protective pigment, is our skin's natural defense against sun exposure.

There are three types of skin cancer:

- Basal cell carcinoma
- Squamous cell carcinoma
- Malignant melanoma

Basal cell cancer is caused by cumulative sun exposure.

Squamous cell cancer is also directly linked to cumulative sun exposure, though it is not as prevalent as basal cell cancer. Squamous cell cancer can migrate, or metastasize, if left untreated. However, the cure rates are around 99 percent.

Melanoma is the most dangerous form of skin cancer. Mainly a disease of white populations, it can readily metastasize. Melanomas occur five times more frequently on the face (perhaps because the facial skin is often exposed, and because it is thinner and more delicate). The risk of melanoma is higher in people who get exposed to the sun intermittently. For example, people who try to get a dark tan in two weeks but get a lobster-red burn instead are more prone to melanoma. People who do not tan easily are also at risk.

This a vital lesson: Early sunburns predispose a child to a dramatically increased risk of melanoma later in life.

A note about preventing children's sun exposure. Wetsuit manufacturers produce a number of kinds of rash guards. Rash guards are lightweight, water-repelling garments designed to prevent rashes resulting from skin rubbing on the inside of a wetsuit. These come in short- and long-sleeve versions, and in a variety of children's sizes. A long-sleeved rash guard is a much better alternative for reducing sun exposure in children than using sunscreen. The rash guard protects skin all day except on the face, hands, and legs, where sunscreen needs to be reapplied.

WAVELENGTH REGIONS OF ULTRAVIOLET (UV) LIGHT			
REGION	WAVELENGTH	OZONE FILTERING	CANCER RISK
UV-A	320–400 nm	Ozone blocks little	Not as dangerous
UV-B	280–320 nm	Ozone blocks most	Most dangerous
UV-C	less than 290 nm	Ozone blocks all	No exposure

ANTICANCER AGENTS FOR SKIN CANCER

vitamin E—both vitamin E and beta carotene protect from melanoma

beta carotene

zinc

antioxidant vitamins such as vitamin C and selenium

low-fat diet decreases basal and squamous skin cancers

avoidance of sunburn, which reduces risk of the most deadly melanoma

avoidance of exposure, especially in the first decade of life, to prevent later development of melanoma

increased DNA repair— sunlight causes errors in DNA, and compounds vital for DNA repair protect against skin cancer

green tea, extracts protect from UV-B induced skin tumors

glutathione, a critical component to guard against UV-A and UV-B

onions and garlic protect from chemically induced skin cancer

It is interesting to note that tanning salons promote the use of UV-B as safe, when it is actually the most dangerous wavelength of ultraviolet light!

Skin Cancer Risk Factors

- Sun-intensive exposures (a sunburn at any time of life increases risk of melanoma, especially before age two)
- Lifetime sun exposure (increases risk of basal and squamous cell cancers)
- Alcohol intake
- Immune system suppression (agents such as AIDS virus or PCBs, which weaken the immune system are likely to increase the risk of melanoma)
- Hair dye (linked to melanoma)
- Freckles (also linked to melanoma)
- Number of moles or birthmarks is a strong predictor for melanoma (any mole larger in diameter than a pencil eraser or with irregular surfaces or coloring is a concern)
- Cigarette smoking (linked to squamous cell skin cancer)
- Chemical exposure (substances in chimney soot, coal tars, pitch, asphalt, creosotes, paraffin waxes, lubricating oils, cutting oils, arsenic, and psoralens are linked with skin cancer)
- People who sunburn easily

Bladder Cancer

Globally a tenfold variation exists for bladder cancer. Some of the highest rates are found in Italy; some of the lowest are in Asia (particularly India and the Philippines). Cancer of the bladder is mostly found in white men. And men as a group are three times more likely to contract this cancer than women.

Bladder Cancer Risk Factors

- Cigarette smoking (smokers pass toxic compounds—mutagens—in their urine)
- High-fat and high-cholesterol diets
- Fried foods (those who consume high levels of fried and charbroiled foods also pass more toxic agents in their urine)
- High pork and beef intake
- Hair dyes (components linked with bladder cancer)
- Chlorinated drinking water (associated with bladder cancer)
- High iron stores (strongly linked to esophagus and bladder cancer)
- Occupation (painters, those who work with aluminum, rubber, leather, and dyestuffs have increased risk of bladder cancer)

ANTICANCER AGENTS FOR BLADDER CANCER

natural and synthetic retinoids

vitamin A foods—associated with less bladder cancer

high vegetable and fruit intake

selenium

foods that increase GST—deficiency predisposes some to bladder cancer

Lymph Cancer

Rates of lymph cancer are higher in industrialized countries than other parts of the world. Non-Hodgkin's lymphoma is a series of cancers that start in the white blood cells, the body's infection-fighting lymph system. In the United States and many other industrialized countries, the incidence of non-Hodgkin's type lymphoma has mushroomed since the 1940s.

A note concerning lymph cancer: Compounds associated with industry are linked to lymph cancer, including PCBs, dioxin, and phenoxy herbicides. These are found in higher levels in meat, fish, dairy, and poultry from industrialized countries. A reduction in these food types will probably result in reduced risk of lymph cancer. Consumption of organic fruits and vegetables will also protect against risk.

Lymphoma Cancer Risk Factors

- Herbicides (risk for lymphoma results from exposure to the herbicides, 4, 5-T—banned in the U.S.—and 2,4-D, a popular chemical for weed control)

- PCBs (can inhibit the immune system and are linked to a rise in lymph cancers)

- Epstein-Barr virus (the virus plus high levels of PCBs produce a level of lymph cancer twenty-two times higher than average)

- Organochlorines (dioxins, for example, are potent immune system poisons linked to lymph cancers)

- Immune system suppression (creates a higher risk of lymph cancer)

- Medication and chemotherapy (drugs to treat epilepsy such as Dilantin and cancer chemotherapy increase the risk of lymph cancer)

- Dairy products

- Hair dyes

- Cigarette smoke

ANTICANCER AGENTS FOR LYMPHOMA

whole grain bread, pasta

organic foods

vegetarian diet

diet low in immune system poisons

Pancreatic Cancer

The pancreas, a small gland located near the small intestine, produces a number of substances—most importantly insulin. Pancreas cancer is mercilessly malignant, and one of the most painful of the fatal cancers. Once detected it will kill its host swiftly.

There is great variation in pancreas cancer internationally. The highest rates are found in African-Americans living in California. The lowest rates are in Asia. Pancreas cancer is about 50 percent more common in men than in women, and it has increased three times in the last few decades in the U.S.

Pancreatic Cancer Risk Factors

- Tobacco smoking (cigarette smokers are twice as likely to get cancer of the pancreas)
- High saturated fat intake
- Animal products (meats, grilled meat, beef, bacon, pork, ham, eggs, dairy foods)
- High intake of carbohydrates (increased risk with white bread, rice, and cereals; decreased risk with whole grain breads)
- Pesticides (elevated risks for increased exposures to insect and plant sprays)
- Steroid hormones (male sex hormones have been shown to stimulate the growth of pancreatic cancer)

ANTICANCER AGENTS FOR PANCREAS CANCER

fresh fruits and vegetables—carrots, citrus fruit, crucifers, greens such as spinach, yellow vegetables

calcium

vitamins C and E

vegetable proteins— beans, lentils, peas

carotenoids—lycopene is consistently lower in subjects who eventually develop cancer of the pancreas

selenium

fiber

Leukemia

Behind home accidents, which are the number one cause of death, cancer remains the second most common killer of American children. And the most commonly diagnosed childhood cancer is leukemia. Leukemia is a progressive increase in abnormal white blood cells (called leukocytes), usually found in the blood in elevated numbers. Leukemia is classified according to the dominant cell type present. Therefore, leukemias include a wide and diverse number of subtypes. For decades, exposures to benzene and to radiation have been suggested as causes of leukemia.

Vitamins A and D and cod liver oil (high in vitamins A and D) protects against leukemia.

Leukemia Risk Factors

- Benzene (used in many products, increases risk of leukemia for painters exposed to benzene in paint and for workers who handle rubber, shoe leather, and printing processes)
- Radiation
- Farming (workers exposed to pesticides have high rates of leukemia)

- Processed meats
- Hair dyes (certain components of hair dyes may cause leukemia)

Cancer of the Kidney

Kidney cancer has steadily increased since 1970. Its incidence is highest in France, and lowest in Bombay, India, and Shanghai, China. Cigarette smoking and high meat intakes remain the more well-known risk factors for cancer of the kidney.

ANTICANCER AGENTS FOR KIDNEYS

high intake of vegetables—especially carrots

high intake of fruits

low meat and protein intake

Kidney Cancer Risk Factors

- Cigarette smoke
- Drugs (analgesics such as acetaminophen)
- Commonly used diuretics
- High meat consumption
- High protein intake
- Tea (studies indicate that heavy use of black tea increases the rate of kidney cancer, particularly in women)
- Occupation (those who work with cadmium, asbestos, polycyclic aromatic hydrocarbons, dry cleaning chemicals, and arsenic have high rates of kidney cancer)
- Obesity

Stomach Cancer

Remarkably, stomach cancer is one of the few cancers that has declined in recent years—although variations do exist around the globe. Increased stomach cancer rates are associated with people who eat highly salted and smoked foods. Home refrigeration in most countries has lead to a decreased risk for stomach cancer, because refrigeration allows for increased consumption of fresh produce, with less reliance on salted, smoked, and pickled foods.

Stomach Cancer Risk Factors

- High-salt foods, which injure the lining of the stomach
- Processed, cured, salted, and smoked meats (nitrates are found in smoked, cured meats like bacon and sausage, salt-dried fish, beer, and pickled vegetables)

0

- High-starch foods (potatoes, bread, rice, and pasta)
- Fried foods
- Cigarette smoking (smoke is known to contain the stomach cancer agent nitrate)
- Radiation exposure
- Bacterial infection (*Helicobacter pylori* among others) are involved with stomach ulcers, and cause a much higher risk of stomach cancer.

Liver Cancer

The most common form of liver cancer (hepatocellular carcinoma) has one of the largest variations globally of any major cancer. Liver cancer is rare in the United States and in western Europe, but it is one of the most common cancers in Asia and parts of Africa. Liver cancer is almost always lethal, therefore more preventive measures are required.

Liver Cancer Risk Factors

- Alcohol and liver cirrhosis
- Aflatoxins (both hepatitis B and aflatoxin exposure may increase liver cancer risk by 60 times)
- Steroid hormones
- Vinyl chloride
- Hepatitis B and C virus
- High iron storage in the body
- Obesity
- Occupational exposure (especially in chemical companies such as producers of auto and rubber, pesticides, wood finish, synthetic textiles, and vinyl chloride)

Throat and Larynx Cancer

Throat cancer, or esophageal cancer, is the ninth most common cancer in the world. It is fatal, even in countries with capable medical care. Larynx cancer, which includes

ANTICANCER AGENTS FOR THE STOMACH

fresh fruits, such as oranges and lemons

raw vegetables (tomatoes, celery, squash, eggplant, lettuce, green and yellow vegetables, onions and garlic)

beta carotene

folic acid (folates)

green tea (which blocks the formation of potent stomach-cancer producing chemicals— nitrosamines)

vitamins A, C, and E

ANTICANCER AGENTS FOR LIVER

vitamins C and E

grapefruit, and fresh citrus fruit in general, which contain a flavonoid called naringin that blocks activation of aflatoxin, a potent liver cancer agent, especially useful against hepatitis B

vegetable fiber and fruit

hepatitis B vaccines— chronic hepatitis B infection is associated with up to 80 percent of liver cancer the vocal cords, has been increasing in recent decades, though it is more common in men. Environmental factors such as tobacco and alcohol play a predominate role in throat cancer.

Throat Cancer Risk Factors

- Heavy tobacco use (black tobacco has more cancer risk than blond tobacco)
- High intake of alcohol (hard liquor such as whiskey is probably more potent than wine or beer)
- Chewing tobacco and betel nut (used in many parts of Asia)
- Ingestion of hot foods (can cause thermal irritation and may lead to increased risk of both throat and larynx cancer)
- Pickled vegetables (eating of pickled vegetables during adolescence has been linked to increased risk)
- Moldy foods (linked to throat cancer)
- High intake of barbecued meat
- High iron stores
- Occupation (at risk are people who work near combustion by-products from incinerators, chimney soot, and diesel exhaust)
- Asbestos

Other risk factors. Poor oral hygiene is a risk factor in oral cancer. Mouthwashes high in alcohol content (over 25 percent) are associated with higher oral cancer risk.

Thyroid Cancer

Thyroid cancer is relatively rare. Dietary intake of iodine may play a role in cancer of the thyroid. Hawaii and Iceland have the highest rates of thyroid cancer in the world. Some of the lowest rates are found in Bombay, India; Wales; and Shanghai, China.

ANTICANCER AGENTS FOR THROAT

fresh fruits

raw vegetables—the protection from vegetables is stronger when uncooked

beta carotene—along with retinol, beta carotene may reduce the risk of oral cancer from tobacco and alcohol

folic acid

fish

green vegetables

vitamin A

vitamin C and green tea, effective in protection from nitrosamine formation

vitamin E, which dramatically inhibited oral cancer by 50 percent in humans

vitamin B12

Thyroid Cancer Risk Factors

- Radiation (significant risk follows radiation exposure in childhood)
- Iodine deficiency (both too much and too little iodine can result in thyroid cancer)
- Poultry, cured meat, cheese, butter
- Alcohol consumption

Soft Tissue Cancers

Cancer that occurs in any of the diversity of tissues such as muscle, fat, and blood vessels, fibrous tissue, and other supporting tissues are collectively referred to as soft tissue cancers, or sarcomas. These have also increased in recent decades.

Soft Tissue Cancer Risk Factors

- Radiation. Radiation therapy increases risk of cancer in soft tissues
- Occupational exposure. Herbicides and chlorophenols used in forestry and agriculture, and compounds such as dioxin, vinyl chloride, and arsenic are strong risk factors
- Insecticides. Chlorinated hydrocarbon insecticides in particular are linked to more cancer
- Smokeless tobacco. Chewing tobacco and snuff have been linked to soft tissue cancers in the lung, head, neck, and face
- High intake of dairy products
- High intake of organ meats. Childhood soft tissue cancer was related to diets high in liver, brains, and tongue

Hodgkin's Disease

Hodgkin's disease is a cancer of the immune system. Its cause is likely to involve an infectious agent, such as the Epstein-Barr virus. Incidence of Hodgkin's disease is more common in males than females, and more

ANTICANCER AGENTS FOR THE THYROID

high fruit intake

high vegetable intake—the most consistent protective factor, especially carrots and green vegetables

coffee—may correlate with reduced thyroid cancer risk

iodine

ANTICANCER AGENTS FOR SOFT TISSUE

antioxidant vitamins

whole grain bread, pasta

likely in economically advantaged populations. Studies have reported increased risk for Hodgkin's disease with herbicide and pesticide exposure.

Hodgkin's Disease Risk Factors

- Economic advantage (children from wealthier families are at greater risk—perhaps due to less exposure to the Epstein-Barr virus in early life)
- Epstein-Barr virus
- Occupation (exposure to herbicides, pesticides, organic solvents, phenoxy acids, and chlorophenols)
- Immune system suppression (immune system poisons are likely risk factors)

Cancer of the Nose, Sinus, and Upper Throat

Chemical exposure to occupational agents seem to be at the bottom of most cancers found in the nose and sinus cavity. Cancer of the nose and sinus is rare in the general population, while specific chemical exposures like those from nickel refining often correlate with higher risk.

Nose, Sinus, and Upper Throat Cancer Risk Factors

- Formaldehyde (from insulation, particle board, and carpet adhesives)
- Chromium and nickel
- Wood dust exposure (even from woodworking)
- Leather dust (from shoe making)
- Salted fish and preserved food products
- Airborne particles (from smoke, fumes, dust, and chemicals may create a risk for upper throat cancer)

Bone Cancer

There is not great international variation in incidence rates of bone cancer. The three types of bone cancer are more likely to occur in males. The death rate for cancers of the bone has declined in recent decades. It is important to restrict childhood X-rays and radiation.

Bone Cancer Risk Factors

- Radiation (children are at greatest risk to bone cancer caused by radiation)
- Chemotherapy (children treated for cancer with chemotherapy have almost a five times greater risk of bone cancer)
- Occupational exposure (radium clock dial workers have increased risk of bone cancer)
- Metal implants (those used for hip replacement are often linked to bone cancer and to cancer of the adjacent tissues)

Brain and Nervous System Cancer

Brain tumors are rapidly fatal and have increased in recent years. Brain tumors are high in children under the age of ten; they decline until age twenty-four to twenty-five; then they steadily increase through adulthood. Brain tumors in the elderly are also emerging. The intake of nitrosamines from processed meats is a potent factor in brain cancer. Therefore, the mother's diet, nutrition, and chemical exposure are critical factors in brain tumor risk for children.

Brain, Nervous System Cancer Risk Factors

- Processed meat (including ham, corned beef, bacon, and cheese, pickled foods, and vegetable fats used in deep frying)
- Head trauma
- Nitrosamines (nitrite and nitrate sources include cured meat, tobacco smoke, cosmetics, automobile interiors, baby pacifiers, and rubber bottle nipples)
- Radiation (though controversial, studies suggest increased brain cancer risk for those in occupations involving electricity and electromagnetic fields)
- Pesticides, herbicides, and insecticides (pesticides, flea collars, pet shampoos, and herbicides may be linked to rising number of childhood brain tumors)

ANTICANCER AGENTS FOR BRAIN, NERVOUS SYSTEM

fresh fruits, which inhibit the formation of cancer producing nitrosamines.

fresh vegetables

vitamins A, C, E, beta carotene and folic acid—children whose mothers took these multivitamin supplements have fewer brain tumors

Nitrosamines

Nitrates are converted into nitrites in the saliva; nitrites are converted into potent cancer-producing nitrosamines in the stomach.

Vegetables contain nitrates too, but in all likelihood these are less available for conversion into nitrites. Vegetables also contain vitamins C and E, which block formation of nitrosamines. Therefore it is likely that fresh fruits and vegetables form less nitrites in the first place, and in the second place they also block the formation of nitrosamines.

This is not the case with processed meats. Intake of nitrosamines from processed meat has also been strongly related to increased nervous system cancers.

Chapter Recap

- A number of cancers can be prevented with specific food regimens.
- Even the most deadly form of skin cancer, melanoma, can be prevented.
- The most consistent pattern for lowering the risk of other cancers is the consumption of fresh fruits and vegetables.
- To reduce cancer overall, it is good to lessen chemical exposure and to limit the amount of processed foods and animal products that are eaten.

Recipes & Menu Ideas

The recipes and menu ideas that follow have been developed over decades in my kitchen, though some are adapted from other health conscious chefs. These cancer-busting diet recommendations will furnish ammunition for warding off cancer and other diseases.

The discovery of a new dish is more beneficial to humanity than the discovery of a new star.
—Anthelme Brillat-Savarin, 1755–1826

Sensible eating has another important advantage: It gives you an overall feeling of "wellness," since you're eating healthful foods that work for rather than against you.

This chapter is divided into two parts. The first contains suggestions for ways to adapt foods right off supermarket shelves, especially helpful for busy households and those with young children. The second part provides a series of cancer-busting recipes.

Simple and Fast Menu Ideas

Prepared tomato sauces can be added to pasta, rice, or rice and beans. Boost protection by adding other cancer blockers, such as fresh shallots, onions, garlic, or vegetable mixes (fresh or frozen). Top with low-fat varieties of parmesan or romano cheese. If possible, do not use canned foods since many are overcooked and contain high levels of sodium.

Bottled or dry soups are okay. Many soups are made from low-fat and low-sodium vegetable stocks. By adding soy products and fresh garlic, you're including cancer deterrents in the time it takes to heat the soup.

Frozen dinners can easily be rendered more healthful. The most common frozen pizzas, burritos, enchiladas, sandwiches, and dinners can all be made more cancer-hindering by adding fresh ginger, turmeric, garlic, onions, salsa, more vegetables, nuts, or fruit.

For rice-based dishes, add a hearty salsa or Chinese vegetables, chicken, and soy products, and perhaps serve them with additional steamed brown or white rice.

What you include in your diet can add years to your life by changing your prospects for cancer. Use the following food list to create your own favorite choices for a personal cancer-hindering diet using the bases of pasta, rice, rice and beans, or soup stocks.

The Super Eight Food Groups

1. *Onion Group*
   garlic, chives, onions, leeks, asparagus, shallots, scallions

2. *Cruciferous group*
   broccoli, collards, Chinese cabbage, cabbage, mustard greens, turnips, cauliflower, bok-choy, radishes, Brussels sprouts, rutabaga, watercress, kale, kohlrabi, garden cress

3. *Nuts and Seeds Group*
   walnuts, pine nuts, pistachios, flaxseed, sesame seeds, almonds, pecans, pumpkin seeds

4. *Grass Group*
   corn, oats, rice, wheat

5. *Legume Group*
   soybeans, green beans, wax beans, peas

6. *Fruit Group*
   oranges, apples, grapes (red and Concord), grapefruit, raspberries, watermelon, tangerines, blackberries, cantaloupe, lemons, strawberries, pineapple, limes, blueberries, honeydew melon

7. *Solanace Group*
   tomatoes, potatoes, sweet potatoes, beets

8. *Umbelliferous Group*
   carrots, parsnips, celeriac, celery, anise, angelica root, parsley, coriander, cumin, dill, lovage, caraway, chervil

Other Important Foods
Cucumber, pumpkin, squash, lettuce, spinach, green and red pepper, spices, turmeric, ginger, seaweed.

Although you may need to take some time learning to prepare meals that include the Super Eight Food Groups, it will be time well spent.

Cancer-Busting Recipes

Spaghetti Squash Stuffed with Spicy Tomato Sauce and Cheese

2 spaghetti squash

1 teaspoon olive oil

32 ounces tomato paste

4 cloves of garlic, minced

4 ounces low-fat cheese

Preheat oven to 375 degrees. Split the squash in half lengthwise and roast for 40 to 50 minutes on a lightly oiled (olive oil) baking sheet. Make a spicy tomato sauce from scratch, or use a prepared variety.

When the squash is tender, spoon the insides to separate the squash into spaghetti-like noodles and add tomato sauce, minced garlic, and cheese. Usually there is enough room in the squash shell to add the sauce; if not, add the excess to a baking dish. Broil in ovenproof cookware until the cheese melts. Serves 4.

Zucchini Lasagna with Soy

3 onions, chopped

4 cloves garlic, minced.

32 ounces tomato sauce

1 16-ounce package lasagna noodles

1 tablespoon basil

1 tablespoon oregano

1/2 tablespoon marjoram

10.5 ounces tofu (firm)

1 pound low-fat mozzarella cheese

2 zucchini, sliced

Preheat oven to 375 degrees. To prepare tomato sauce: In a large pan lightly cook onions and garlic in a small amount of sesame oil. Add a prepared 32 ounces of tomato sauce (or make by adding 4 ounces of tomato paste to 28 ounces of chopped Italian tomatoes). Mix all spices into the sauce and bring to a boil, then quickly turn to simmer. Boil lasagna noodles. Cut the tofu into thin slices, and use it in place of ricotta cheese. To assemble the lasagna: alternate layers of noodles, sliced zucchini squash, tofu, sauce, and cheese. Oven-bake for 40 minutes. Serves 4 to 6.

Stuffed Peppers

1/2 cup rice

1 cup walnuts

1 medium onion, chopped

8 cloves garlic, minced

1/2 cup pasta sauce, spiced

1 teaspoon basil

1 tablespoon Worcestershire sauce

3 green bell peppers, cut lengthwise

1 can (15 ounces) tomato sauce

Cook rice. Chop walnuts and onions, press garlic and add to pasta sauce while simmering. Add Worcestershire sauce and fresh spices (if possible), to taste. Finally, mix rice with sauce and fill peppers. Microwave on medium-high for 20 to 25 minutes. Serves 4 to 6.

Fettuccine with Broccoli and Tomatoes

12 ounces fettuccine

3 cups broccoli cut florets

2 cups sundried tomatoes

3 cloves garlic, minced

3 tablespoons olive or sesame oil

1/2 cup grated Parmesan cheese

Follow the package directions for cooking the fettuccine. Around 3 minutes before the pasta is cooked, add the broccoli to the boiling water; at two minutes before add the sundried tomatoes. Cook until the broccoli is tender but crispy. Do not overcook. Drain water and toss fettuccine together with vegetables, minced garlic, and oil. Sprinkle cheese on top. Serves 4 to 6.

Italian Ziti Bake

1 pound ziti, rigatoni, or bow-tie pasta

1 teaspoon sesame oil

5 cloves fresh garlic, minced

1 to 2 red onions, chopped

3 zucchini, diced

1/2 teaspoon each oregano and basil

1/4 teaspoon ground red pepper

2 egg whites

10.5 ounces tofu (soft)

1 can (28 ounces) crushed tomatoes

3/4 cup low-fat mozzarella cheese

1/4 cup grated Parmesan cheese

Preheat oven to 350 degrees. Cook pasta partially so that the inside is slightly uncooked. While pasta is cooking, heat the sesame oil in a saucepan on low heat and add the garlic, onions, and zucchini. Cook, covered, until the vegetables are soft but still crispy. Add spices and simmer for 10 minutes. Blend together the egg whites and tofu. Lightly smear a film of sesame oil inside a large casserole pan. Layer the pasta between the egg white-tofu blend and crushed tomatoes. Add the mozzarella and parmesan cheese to the top and bake until they turn a hint of golden color, about 40 minutes. Serves 4 to 6.

Mexican-style Fresh Tomato Pasta

1 pound bow-tie pasta

2 cups chopped tomatoes

1/3 cup red onion, sliced

1 can (4 ounces) chopped green chilies

1/3 cup chopped cilantro

1/4 cup olive or sesame oil

2 tablespoons fresh lime juice

4 cloves pressed garlic

Cook pasta according to instructions. Add all sauce ingredients together in a large bowl. Add hot pasta to bowl and toss with other ingredients. Serves 4 to 6.

Walnut Pesto with Acorn Squash

4 acorn squash

1 teaspoon sesame oil

For pesto:

4 tablespoons chopped walnuts

4 cloves garlic

1 cup fresh parsley

4 tablespoons fresh sage

1/3 teaspoon freshly ground pepper

3 tablespoons sesame oil

4 tablespoons vegetable broth

Preheat oven to 375 degrees. Cut squash lengthwise into two equal parts and remove seeds. Place squash with cut side down on a baking sheet that has been lightly oiled with sesame oil and bake for 30 to 40 minutes, or until tender.

To prepare the pesto: Lightly toast the walnuts in a small saucepan for a few minutes and remove from heat. In a blender or food processor add garlic, parsley, sage, pepper, and nuts. Blend until finely chopped. Add sesame oil and vegetable broth and blend until the pesto has a smooth consistency. Add 2 teaspoons of pesto to each half of the hot squash. Serve remaining pesto in a bowl. Serves 6 to 8.

Lotus Chicken

6 pounds whole roasting chicken

For marinade:

2 tablespoons soy sauce (low salt)

2 tablespoons sesame oil

2 tablespoons rice wine

For stuffing:

    4 dried lotus leaves

    3 large dried black mushrooms

    1 tablespoon sesame oil

    1/2 cup watercress

    1/2 cup water chestnuts

    1/2 cup bamboo shoots, chopped

    8 scallions, chopped

    1/2 cup lotus seeds

    1 tablespoon soy sauce (low-salt)

    2 tablespoons rice wine

Preheat oven to 350 degrees. Soak lotus leaves in hot water for 30 minutes. Soak dried mushrooms for 15 minutes; dry then chop. Mix marinade ingredients and evenly coat the chicken with the marinade. In a hot wok or skillet, add the sesame oil and lightly stir-fry all the vegetables for the stuffing and add the soy sauce and rice wine. Stuff the chicken and close the cavity. Bake 45 minutes, together with remaining stuffing, covered. Uncover for the last 5 minutes. Note: Lotus leaves and seeds can be obtained from Asian food stores. Serves 6 to 8.

Cancer-Nipping Salads and Side Dishes

Chinese Chicken Salad

4 tablespoons sesame oil

6 tablespoons rice vinegar

2 tablespoons soy sauce (low-salt)

6 cloves garlic, minced

1 cup chicken, cut bite size

1/4 cup fresh ginger

1 red bell pepper, diced and roasted

1/2 cup celery, sliced

1/2 cup scallions, sliced

1 cup watercress

10 ounces spinach

1/3 pound snow peas

1 pound bean sprouts

3/4 cup shiitake mushrooms

3/4 cup mandarin oranges

4 tablespoons sesame seeds, toasted

In a blender add sesame oil, rice vinegar, soy sauce, and garlic. Puree. Add the puree to a heated wok and stir-fry together with chicken until cooked. Add ginger, red bell pepper, celery, and scallions and stir-fry for 2 to 3 minutes. Add the remaining ingredients and stir-fry for 1 minute. Sprinkle toasted sesame seeds on top. Serves 6 to 8.

Curried Chicken and Spinach Pasta Salad

3/4 pound pasta shells

3 tablespoons slivered almonds

1 tablespoon Madras curry powder

1/2 cup low-fat yogurt

1/3 cup mango chutney

1 teaspoon turmeric

1/2 tablespoon cayenne pepper

1/4 teaspoon cinnamon

2 cups cooked chicken, cut into cubes

1/2 cup raisins

1/2 cup scallions

1/2 cup celery, diced

10 ounces fresh spinach, torn

Cook pasta al dente (not quite fully cooked) and set aside. In a saucepan, heat almonds over low heat, stirring constantly for a few minutes. Remove almonds to a small bowl to cool. In the same saucepan lightly toast the curry powder and remove from heat. Add low-fat yogurt (or low-fat sour cream), chutney, and spices to a small bowl and mix thoroughly. In a large bowl combine the cooked chicken cubes with raisins, scallions, celery, spinach, and the pasta. Add the yogurt dressing and toss to evenly coat the pasta. Optional: Add more spices to taste. Top with toasted almonds. Serves 4.

Tomato Basil Salad

6 large red or yellow tomatoes

1/4 cup fresh basil

8 ounces low-fat mozzarella cheese

2 teaspoons balsamic vinegar

1/4 cup sesame or olive oil

Cut tomatoes into wedges, tear the basil leaves into bite-size pieces, cube the mozzarella cheese, add to a salad bowl. Mix in the balsamic vinegar and oil and toss. Serves 4.

Chinese Noodle Salad

3/4 pound Chinese noodles

3 tablespoons sesame oil

1 pound broccoli florets

1 red bell pepper, diced

1 pound baby asparagus, cut into bite-size pieces

1/4 cup sesame seeds, toasted

1/3 cup chives, sliced

For dressing:

1/2 cup vegetable stock

1/4 cup red wine vinegar

1/4 cup cooking sherry

2 tablespoons soy sauce

3 tablespoons sesame oil

2 tablespoons Chinese chili sauce

1/4 cup scallions, sliced

1/4 cup fresh ginger

8 cloves garlic

1 cup shiitake mushrooms

In a large pot cook the noodles. Drain, rinse, and toss with 3 tablespoons sesame oil. Steam broccoli, red bell pepper, and asparagus until tender and crispy.

For dressing:

In a medium pan add vegetable stock, vinegar, sherry, soy sauce, sesame oil, chili sauce, scallions, ginger, and garlic. Heat until boiling; then quickly turn heat to low and add mushrooms. Simmer mixture for 2 minutes, stirring constantly. In a large bowl, toss noodles together with the dressing.
Top with toasted sesame seeds and chives. Serves 4 to 6.

Cauliflower and Broccoli Soup

1 1/2 cups red potatoes

3/4 cup cauliflower florets

3/4 cup broccoli florets

2 1/2 cups vegetable stock

1 1/2 cups soy milk

6 cloves garlic, minced

3/4 cup scallions, sliced

6 tablespoons sesame oil

1 teaspoon white pepper

Boil potatoes for 10 minutes and remove from heat. In a medium-size pan combine the vegetables, vegetable stock, and soy milk. Bring to a boil and quickly simmer for a few minutes. Drain potatoes and cut into small pieces; add to soup. In a small saucepan sauté the garlic and scallions in sesame oil. Serve warm with white pepper sprinkled on top. Serves 4.

Miso Soup

There are a number of instant soups that only require the addition of hot water. Choose brands lowest in sodium.

Spicy Four-Bean Chili

4 ounces black beans

4 ounces kidney beans

4 ounces pinto beans

4 ounces brown lentils

1 teaspoon cumin seeds

1 teaspoon coriander seed

2 carrots, diced

1 red bell pepper, sliced

3 stalks celery, sliced

8 ounces mushrooms, diced

2 red onions, chopped

8 cloves garlic, minced

4 ounces tomato paste

14 ounces chopped tomatoes

4 fresh chili peppers

1 tablespoon chili powder

1/2 teaspoon ground cumin

1 teaspoon black pepper

1 tablespoon sesame oil

2 pints vegetable broth

Soak dry beans in water overnight (lentils do not need to be soaked). Discard water and cook beans in fresh water until soft, around 2 hours. Heat sesame oil and lightly cook onion and garlic. Add the cumin and coriander seed, and cook on low heat until the seeds begin to pop open. Mix in the vegetables, tomato paste, chopped tomatoes, lentils, and beans with chilies and spices. Bring the mixture to a boil, then simmer on very low heat for 1 hour or longer. Add more vegetable stock if necessary and season to taste. Serves 6.

Zesty Tomato Tofu Soup

1 small red onion

1 can tomato soup

1 bay leaf

8 ounces of tofu (firm), diced

1 teaspoon basil

1/2 teaspoon oregano

1/2 teaspoon cayenne pepper

Add all ingredients to soup pot. Bring the mixture to a quick boil, then simmer on very low heat while adding spices. Add more vegetable stock if necessary and season to taste. Serves 2.

Quick Cancer-Annihilating Breakfasts

Italian Omelet

2 teaspoons sesame oil

2 medium red onions, chopped

4 cloves garlic, minced

1/2 teaspoon oregano

1/4 teaspoon rosemary

1/2 teaspoon basil

1/2 teaspoon thyme

1/2 teaspoon freshly ground pepper

24 small asparagus spears, cut bite size

1 green bell pepper, diced

1 yellow bell pepper, diced

1 red bell pepper, diced

8 egg whites (or egg substitute)

8 ounces fat-free cheddar cheese

4 green onions, sliced

Preheat broiler. In an ovenproof skillet heat the sesame oil with onions and garlic. Cook for 3 minutes. Add spices, asparagus, and bell peppers to the skillet and lightly cook for another 3 minutes. In a large bowl beat egg whites and pour over vegetables. Top with cheddar cheese (or another low-fat cheese) and green onions and place the skillet under the broiler. Broil for 5 to 10 minutes, or until the cheese melts. Be careful not to overcook. For a spicy version add jalapeño peppers. Serves 6 to 8.

Cinnamon-Apple Oat Bran Cereal

1 cup uncooked oat bran cereal

1 teaspoon vanilla

1/2 cup raisins

1/4 cup applesauce

1 teaspoon cinnamon

Optional: apple slices, bananas, fresh fruit

2 cups skim milk

In a large pan bring water to a boil and slowly stir in oat bran. Follow oat bran package directions for water quantity. Stir oat bran constantly until the water starts to boil again, then reduce heat to simmer. Mix in vanilla, raisins, and applesauce and cook for an additional 2 minutes. Top with slices of fresh apple, cinnamon, and bananas, or your favorite fruit. Add soy milk or skim milk. Serves 4.

Scrambled Soy Omelet

10.5 ounces tofu (firm)

3 tablespoons sesame oil

1/2 cup broccoli, florets

1/2 cup cauliflower, florets

1 red bell pepper, chopped

4 green onions, chopped

1 grated carrot

1 pint cherry tomatoes

1 teaspoon cayenne

1 teaspoon turmeric

1 teaspoon black pepper

1/2 cup low-fat cheese

Drain the tofu and mash into small pieces. Preheat broiler. On moderate heat, add sesame oil to an ovenproof skillet. Add broccoli, cauliflower, and red bell pepper, and lightly cook for 3 minutes. Add tofu together with some of the green onions, the carrot, tomatoes, and spices. Add sufficient cayenne and turmeric to give the tofu an attractive color. Season the top with the same spices and remaining green onions to taste. Top with low-fat cheese and broil until the cheese melts. Serves 4 to 6.

Muesli Pancakes with Fresh Fruits

3/4 cup Muesli cereal

1/4 cup whole wheat flour

2 teaspoons baking powder

1 cup skim milk

2 tablespoons honey

2 slightly beaten egg whites

1/2 cup pecans, chopped

1/2 teaspoon vanilla

2 tablespoons sesame oil

For berry sauce:

12 ounces frozen berries

2 tablespoons honey

Mix dry ingredients and add liquid. Coat griddle with sesame oil and cook pancakes until slightly brown. Use fresh berries for the sauce, and puree in a blender with honey. Use frozen raspberries, blueberries, or blackberries if fresh berries aren't available. (Note: Use aluminum-free baking powder.) Top pancakes with sauce and pecans. Serves 4.

Delicious Cancer-Devouring Desserts

Layered Fruit Salad

2 oranges

3 bananas

4 kiwis

2 apples

2 peaches

1 pound red seedless grapes

1 pint fresh raspberries

1 quart fresh strawberries

1/2 cup freshly squeezed orange juice

juice of 2 lemons

Rinse fruit. Peel and slice oranges, bananas, and kiwis. Slice apples and peaches. Layer fruit with grapes in the bottom followed by bananas, apples, oranges, peaches, raspberries, strawberries. Top with slices of kiwi. Pour fresh squeezed orange juice and lemon juice over the fruit, and serve chilled. Serves 4.

Low-fat Chocolate Mint Brownies

3 egg whites and 1 egg

2 ounces unsweetened chocolate

8 teaspoons fruit juice substitute or sugar

1/4 teaspoon peppermint extract

1/3 cup macadamia oil

1/2 cup flour

1 tablespoon low-fat milk

1/3 cup almonds, chopped

1/3 cup pecans, chopped

Preheat oven to 350 degrees. Beat egg whites and egg until frothy. Heat chocolate, fruit juice substitute (use fructose or sugar but not an artificial sweetener), peppermint, and macadamia oil in a double boiler until melted. Stir the chocolate mixture into the egg mixture and combine flour, milk, and nuts until thoroughly mixed. Add the mixture to a baking pan that has been lightly greased with macadamia nut oil. Bake for about 15 minutes. Serves 4 to 6.

Beverages

Black Tea

black tea

1/3 lemon

3 ounces soy milk

Use Ceylon, Darjeeling, Oolong, flavored or orange pekoe teas. Only add lemon or soy milk to black teas (do not add both). Serve iced or hot.

Green Tea

After boiling allow the water to stand for a few minutes before adding the tea, otherwise it will taste bitter. Also, if you add too much green tea it becomes bitter. Buy bulk green tea (loose tea) from Asian food stores (or mail order, see appendix F) over prepackaged tea in bags. Serve iced or hot.

Fruit Shake with Soy

5 ounces of silken tofu (soft)

8 ounces low-fat yogurt

1 pint strawberries

1 to 2 bananas

Raspberries, blueberries, and other fruits including citrus and melons can be included in this shake. Add tofu to blender with yogurt. Optional: For a dairy-free fruit shake, add tofu only and replace yogurt with additional fruit. Add fresh fruit and blend at high speed for 3 minutes or until fruit is blended evenly. Top with sliced banana and berries. Serves 2.

Other Beverage Ideas

Good beverages include fermented ginger ales, fruit juices, orange and grapefruit juices. You can also blend fruit juice with sparkling mineral water for a refreshing drink. Also try light red wines, especially from California, since these wines have low amounts of lead compared to Italian red wines.

As you introduce more and more cancer-hampering foods into your cooking, you will develop your own recipes, as well as learn variations and new ideas from friends.

Chapter Recap

- A number of simple, fast chemopreventive menus can come right off the grocery shelf.
- By eating soy, fresh garlic, green tea, and other foods from the Super Eight Food Groups, you are benefiting from nature's best cancer deterrents.

Author Afterword

All of us are rightfully concerned about cancer. And precious few of us are cloistered monks. To the contrary, we live in a very real world of fast foods, hectic schedules, cigarette smoking, smog, and pesticides. In short, we are besieged by cancer-causing agents.

The purpose of this book is not to make everyone an overnight vegetarian; frankly, that would be downright impractical. Rather, the purpose of my research and writing is to give real-world readers like you options for coexistence in a society overwhelmed by cancer. And, this book represents hope for the future—while, at the same time, recognizing that all of us are simply human beings looking for a better life for ourselves and our children.

The simple messages in this book are: Cancer detection will never be as effective as cancer prevention; more than 80% of all known cancers can be prevented; a cancer-busting regimen requires whole fresh foods; we are what we eat; and, most importantly, we can win the struggle against cancer if we eat to beat cancer.

Absolute scientific proof that may be a lifetime in coming, is better left to scientists. In the real world, we cannot wait for researchers to bless everything, lest death overtake us.

Knowledge and information replace fear; options empower us; and action will change not only our lives but the lives of generations to come.

Nothing on earth will be more fulfilling than to level cancer at one swoop and get our lives where they belong—where they were over a century ago—a society where cancer is rare.

Appendix A

Scientific Support for This Book

We are flooded with new information every day concerning diet and cancer. As a critical thinking adult, how do you make sense of it? A critical thinker by definition is someone who can think objectively and fairly about the ideas and views he or she believes in, as well as opposing ideas and views. A critical thinker is not swayed by media coverage and is able to suspend judgment on a controversial issue until the information necessary to make a decision has been gathered. But how long can you afford to suspend judgment without having your health suffer? Tapping into the vast scientific literature can be daunting for someone who is not a scientist.

Eat to Beat Cancer has done the work for you by completing a rigorous literature search and translating highly technical journal articles into usable information. The scientific studies on which *Eat to Beat Cancer* is based show a high level of confirmation for chemoprevention, the idea that health can be achieved through a cancer-busting prevention diet.

1. Well over 200 human studies have examined the association between fruit and vegetable intake and cancers of the lung, colon, breast, cervix, esophagus, oral cavity, stomach, bladder, pancreas, and ovary.
2. When the studies were analyzed by statistical methods, the significant protective effect of fruits and vegetables was identified in well over 80 percent of the dietary studies. People with low fruit and vegetable intake demonstrate about a two times increase in the risk of cancer, compared to those with high intakes. In particular, fruits were shown to be highly protective in over 95 percent of the studies that examined cancer found in the oral cavity, esophagus, and larynx.
3. These dietary intake studies were conducted in almost 20 different nations and include diverse populations from around the globe. It is difficult to imagine a different interpretation of fruit and vegetable intake that could explain identical conclusions among such different groups.

4. In an attempt to be comprehensive, not all the dietary ingredients listed in this book have been proven effective beyond a shadow of a doubt. Some have been associated with less risk in a specific cancer. In fact many of these dietary agents will never be unequivocally proven as cancer preventive. However, since the foods and nutrients are components of a healthful diet, they will not harm you and could be the difference between health and cancer.

(The vast majority of these studies have been published in peer-reviewed journals or reviewed by leading scientists to validate the methods).

Evidence is overwhelming that shows a strong link between fruit and vegetable consumption and prevention of cancer. Further, there are countless animal and experimental studies to support these findings. These are covered in this book.

HUMAN STUDIES OF FRUIT AND VEGETABLE INTAKE AND CANCER PREVENTION[1]			
SITES	NO. OF STUDIES	PROTECTIVE $(P<0.05)$[2]	HARMFUL $(P<0.05)$[2]
All sites	156	128	7
Lung	25	24	0
Larynx	4	4	0
Oral Cavity	9	9	0
Esophagus	16	15	0
Stomach	19	17	1
Colorectal	27	20	3
Bladder	5	3	0
Pancreas	11	9	0
Cervix	8	7	0
Ovary	4	3	0
Breast	14	8	0
Prostate	14	4	2
Miscellaneous	8	6	0

[1] Adapted from Block, G. et al., Fruit, vegetables, and cancer prevention: a review of the epidemiological evidence. *Nutrition and Cancer* (1992)18:1-29.

[2] The p values are a measure of statistical strength or significance for the measured response or test. The smaller the p value the greater the level of statistical significance.

A Note About Animal Studies

Some methods used for cancer testing in animals have received mixed reviews, such as the maximum tolerated dose (MTD). Many scientists bristle at the mention of the MTD: the highest possible dose an animal can tolerate during testing. Scientists who test compounds for cancer administer test compounds at the maximum tolerated doses. MTD critics contend that when animals are faced with such high doses of chemicals, the normal protective systems are strained, spurring widespread cell death. They claim the increased killing of cells causes cancer. The data supports this claim since about half of tested chemicals (natural and synthetic) cause rodent cancers.

Then there are those who place no usefulness at all in animal studies. Finally there are scientists who will never have enough data to satisfy their curiosity.

This constant debate is nice for scientific forums, but it baffles the average consumer.

We will always need more data, but we must also judiciously use the information that is currently available and take direction from that. So rather then wait for a perfect world, *Eat To Beat Cancer* makes the best use of the most current animal data available regarding eating fresh, healthy foods.

Appendix B

Nutritional Quackery

The American College of Physicians defines medical quackery as "the promotion and commercialization of unproven and potentially dangerous health products and procedures."

Present laws do not stop the flood of deceptive, false, and misleading nutritional claims that appear everywhere. The current law only requires that misleading health claims not appear on the label of the product.

Sometimes quackery is easy to identify. The following points will assist you in identifying false nutritional claims.

Red Flags

1. "Miracle cure"
2. "Cure alls" promoted as curing multiple ailments
3. Personal testimonials as proof
4. "Ancient, Exotic, Prehistoric, Special, Secret Formula"
5. Available exclusively from only one supplier
6. Too good to be true, or promises rapid or dramatic results
7. "Overlooked by the medical community"
8. Has logic but no scientific evidence to support its claims
9. Boasts endorsers with questionable credentials
10. Sources uncited or questionable scientific sources for the health benefits being promoted

The greater the number of these red flags that pop up when you evaluate questionable nutritional claims, the less likely it is that the claims are valid.

Nutritional fraud is flourishing in the United States. The federal government needs to take a more active role in monitoring this multibillion dollar industry. In the meantime, buyer beware—some products are dangerous to your health.

Herbal products are not tested for safety or effectiveness. Teas and capsules are a form of herbal remedies, and many herbal products and teas are toxic! Do not take any product that contains comfrey, which is toxic to the liver and has been banned in Canada, but regrettably, not in the United States.

Appendix C

Twenty-Three Ways Off the Pesticide Treadmill

1. Use beneficial insects in your yard and garden, or insects that prey on pest insects, such as lacewings, ladybug beetles, predatory mites, parasitic wasps, and spiders.

2. To support beneficial insects, grow plants such as white lace flower, clover, evening primrose, cilantro, fennel, caraway, dill, flowering buckwheat, white yarrow, and tansy.

3. Place flea traps near where your pet sleeps and use flea combs. Bathe pets often with mild shampoos.

4. Use flea traps that attract fleas to a light and trap them on sticky paper. Or place a shallow bowl filled with soapy water in front of a night light.

5. In pet bedding use eucalyptus, rosemary, and bay leaves to deter fleas.

6. Use supplements (garlic, sulfur, and zinc) that help repel fleas, such as the product Pet Guard™.

7. In homes block the entry of ants with duct tape or petroleum jelly, or use Tanglefoot™.

8. Pour boiling water down ant colonies and nests you want to destroy.

9. Wash ant-infested surfaces with soap and water to remove the chemical trails left by ants that lead them to food.

10. Baits such as Drax™ Ant Kill Gel limits the exposure to humans, pets, and the environment. Ants eat the bait and take it back to the colony where it is shared. Baits are the best way to kill the egg-laying queen.

11. Deny ants food and water. Store dry foods in airtight containers or in the refrigerator. To protect pet food from ants, place the food bowl inside a larger bowl filled with water to create a water barrier around the food.

12. Sapsuckers are common garden pests that suck sap from plants and include: aphids, mealybugs, scale, whiteflies, spider mites, and leafhoppers. Use a strong water spray to physically remove sapsuckers.

13. To control sapsuckers use petroleum jelly and detergent to create nontoxic sticky traps or buy TackTrap™.

14. To kill sapsuckers prune heavily infested areas of the plant and then spray with or submerge in soapy water.

15. Caterpillars and cutworms: Hand removal is the most effective for small numbers.

16. Caterpillars and cutworms: Make a neem oil extract trap. Neem tree oil is effective when caterpillars contact or eat treated plants. Safer Bio-Neem™ contains neem oil.

17. Caterpillars and cutworms: Protect seedlings with seedling stems, paper collars, or cone-shaped screening.

18. Caterpillars and cutworms: Use natural enemies or beneficial insects.

19. Powdery mildew and rust: To reduce the spread of infection, remove infected plant parts as they appear.

20. Powdery mildew and rust: In January, prune your roses back and remove all leaves and leaf litter at the base of the plants. This drastically cuts down on the over-wintering spores.

21. Hand weeding is best for home gardening. It is easiest to remove the weeds while they are seedlings. Handheld cultivators are good to cut down the weeds before they go to flower, preventing seed dispersal.

22. You can use a propane torch to flame the weeds. The flame should be held five inches above the weed for 10 to 15 seconds.

23. You can use the sun to kill weeds. Apply a 2-millimeter, clear plastic tarp over weed-infested area. Be sure to flatten the weeds and seal the edges with soil or rocks to retain heat. Remove after 3 to 4 weeks.

See appendix F for product sources.

Appendix D
Lead in Calcium Supplements

As shocking as it may seem, most major brands of calcium supplements and antacids contain significant levels of lead. This was recently revealed by a group of organizations including the Natural Resources Defense Council, Alliance to End Childhood Lead Poisoning, Physicians for Social Responsibility, and the Sierra Club. Dr. Russell Flegal conducted the analysis at the University of California, Santa Cruz, Department of Environmental Toxicology.

Currently the manufacturing practices of calcium supplements and antacids are largely unregulated. Tragically, consumers are unknowingly exposed to unacceptable levels of lead through the routine ingestion of calcium supplements. For further information contact the Natural Resources Defense Council (see appendix G).

Calcium Supplements
The calcium products listed below have the lowest levels of lead and also meet the requirements of California Proposition 65.

CALCIUM SUPPLEMENTS		
Product Name	Calcium Per Tablet (miligrams)	Lead Content (micrograms)[1]
Posture-D High Potency Calcium with Vitamin D (Whitehall Laboratories, Inc.)	600 mg	0.2 to 0.5
Tums 500 Calcium Supplement, Chewable (SmithKline Beecham)	500 mg	0.3 to 0.4

[1] Lead content per minimum and maximum dose.

Antacids
The antacid products listed below have the lowest levels of lead and also meet the requirements of California Proposition 65.

ANTACIDS		
Product Name	Calcium Per Tablet (miligrams)	Lead Content (micrograms)[1]
Children's Mylanta Chewable Antacid, Fruit Punch and Bubble Gum Flavors (Johnson and Johnson-Merck)	160 mg	0.1 to 0.2
Children's Mylanta Liquid Antacid, Fruit Punch and Bubble Gum Flavors (Johnson and Johnson-Merck)	160 mg	0.03 to 0.2

[1] Lead content per minimum dose. Do not exceed dosage information from the manufacturer.

Appendix E

Eleven Ways to Eliminate Aluminum Exposure

1. Do not use aluminum cookware, especially with high-acid foods.

2. Cut down on table salt, which contains aluminum.

3. Limit non-dairy creamers.

4. Watch out for antacids, since many upset stomach remedies have high aluminum contents.

5. Limit baking soda (reduce acid foods since more aluminum is absorbed).

6. Reduce dietary supplements that use aluminum as a binding agent.

7. Drink bottled water.

8. Reduce uptake of aluminum by increasing calcium foods.

9. Reduce intake of baked goods unless ingredients include a non-aluminum baking soda.

10. Increase silicon intake since it reduces uptake and removal of aluminum. Dietary sources include: unrefined grains, cereal products, and root vegetables.

11. Reduce processed breakfast cereals.

Appendix F
Better Brands

Don't have time to shop for organic foods? Buy them through the mail from mail-order companies.

Mail Order Organic Foods

Good Eats
P.O. Box 756
Richboro, PA 18954-0756
(800) 490-0044 or (215) 674-2217
Fax (215) 443-7087
E-mail: goodeats@voicenet.com
http://www.hlthmall.com/healthmall/goodeats/
Offers more than 2,000 natural foods items from some of the industry's best-known names.

The Gourmet Food Store
P.O. Box 524
Lake Bluff, IL 60044
(847) 244-9595
Fax (708) 622-8893
E-mail: gourmetstore@sendit.com
http://www.gourmetstore.com
Specializes in gourmet items, especially unusual and hard-to-locate dried items.

Harvest Direct
PO Box 988
Knoxville, TN 37901-0988
(800) 835-2867

The Mail Order Catalog
PO Box 180
Summertown, TN 38483
(800) 695-2241

Walnut Acres Organic Farms
Penns Creek, PA 17862-0800
(800) 433-3998 (24 hours a day, 7 days a week)
http://walnutacres.com
Has many organic foods including beef and hot dogs.

Dixie Diner's Club
7800 Amelia
Houston, TX 77055
(713) 688-4993

Eden Foods, Inc.
701 Tecumseh Road
Clinton, MI 49236
(517) 456-7424

Natural Lifestyle
16 Lookout Drive
Asheville, NC 28804
(800) 752-2775

Organic Swiss Chocolate (Rapunzel)
Mercantile Food Company
P O Box SS
Ghent, NY 12565
(518) 672-0190

Mail-Order Vitamins and Supplements

L&H Vitamins
32-33 47th Avenue
Long Island City, New York 11101
(800) 221-1152 (10 PM, EST)
Fax (718) 361-1437
http://www.lhvitamins.com
A discount supplier of top-quality product lines.

Vitamin Research Products, Inc.
3579 Hwy 50 East
Carson City, NV 89701
(800) 877-2447 (24 hours)
http://www.vrp.com
Lycopene supplements

Fruit and Vegetable Wash

Organiclean ™
Walnut Acres (see Mail-Order Organic Foods)
(800) 433-3998

Citri-Glow
MIA Rose Products Inc.
Costa Mesa, CA 92626
(800) 292-6339
A citrus based all-purpose cleaner

Pesticide Alternatives (found at garden stores)

Tanglefoot ™

Pet Guard ™

TackTrap ™

Drax ™

Bio-Neem ™

Suppliers of Beneficial Insects

Bio-Integral Resource Center
PO Box 7414
Berkeley, CA 94707
(510) 524-2567

Gardens Alive!
5100 Schenley Place
Lawrenceberg, IN
(812) 537-8650

Peaceful Valley Farm Supply
PO Box 2209
Grass Valley, CA 95945
(916) 272-4769

Ricon Vitova Beneficial Insectaries
PO Box 1555
Ventura, CA 93002
(805) 643-5407

Island Seed and Feed
29 S. Fairview
Goleta, CA 93117
(805) 967-5262

Trace Metal Analysis of Hair Samples

Biochemical Laboratories
PO Box 157
Edgewood, NM
(800) 545- 6562

Personal Air Filter Face Masks

Reduce exercise-induced asthma, prevent asthma, and dust, particulate, and environmental pollutant exposures with an air filter face mask.

Greenscreen Air Filter Face Masks
3145 Geary Blvd., Suite 108
San Francisco, CA 94118
(415) 387-3800
E-mail: http://www.greenscreen@castleweb.com
httl://www. castleweb.com/~grnscrn

Lead Check Kits

Lead Check Swabs
HybriVet Systems, Inc.
PO Box 1210
Framingham, MA 01701
(800) 262-LEAD

WaterTest Corporation
New London, New Hampshire
(603) 526-6756
Water quality test for lead.

Appendix G
Internet Resources: From Cancer to Nutrition

Breast Cancer

The Public Health Institute's Breast Cancer Answers Project
Their mission is to improve access to, and awareness of, breast cancer clinical trial information, to support patients receiving treatment, and to improve the quality of life for patients with breast cancer.
http://www.canceranswers.org

Breast CancerNet
This is a nonprofit clearinghouse, which has the latest news and articles on breast cancer, as well as hundreds of links to other breast cancer-related sites and resources on the Internet.
http://www.breastcancer.net/bcn.html

Breast Cancer Information Clearinghouse
Information for breast cancer patients and their families. It is maintained as a partnership of organizations that provide information about cancer to the public.
http://nysernet.org/bcic

Breast Cancer Information Service
The Breast Cancer Information Service provides useful information to people seeking information about diagnosis, treatment, prevention, support, and insurance issues concerning breast cancer.
http://trfn.clpgh.org/bcis/ (semi-retired)

Breast Cancer Information Center
This site has general information on breast cancer, mammography, and support groups. They also have a great list of ongoing clinical trials.
http://www.feminist.org/other/bc/bchome.html

Beth Israel Guide to Breast Cancer
Information on treatment options.
http://www.bimc.edu/netscape2/breastcancer/intro.html
http://www.bidmc.harvard.edu/breastcare/

UCLA MedNET
This is part of the UCLA breast cancer patient learning series.
http://www.mednet.ucla.edu/healthtopics/PLS/breast.htm

NHRC (National Breast Cancer Centre)
Australian government site,
http://www.nbcc.org.au/

Breast Cancer Detection

Breast Self-Examination (Sloan-Kettering Cancer Center)
http://www.mskcc.org/document/pedbse.htm

NCI Breast Cancer Prevention
Information on breast cancer risks, menopausal hormonal replacement therapy.
http://nci.nih.gov/

National Institute of Cancer
A service of the National Cancer Institute for people with cancer, their families, doctors, nurses, and other health care professionals.
(See above address)

Prostate Cancer

OncoLink Prostate Cancer
http://oncolink.upenn.edu/disease/prostate/index.html

The University of Michigan Prostate Cancer Home Page
http://www.cancer.med.umich.edu/prostcan/prostcan.html

Prostate Cancer InfoLink
http://www.comed.com/Prostate

Prostate Cancer: FAQs
http://www.comed.com/Prostate

Prostate Cancer Home Page—University of Michigan Prostate Cancer Home Page
http://www.cancer.med.umich.edu/prostcan/prostcan.html

Prostate Cancer
This link is to the National Cancer Institute Information site on prostate cancer. It offers an overview of the disease, as well as information on staging and treatment.
http://cancernet.nci.nih.gov/clinpdq/pif/Prostate_cancer_Patient.html

Prostate Pointers
This is a fairly extensive list of prostate cancer-related Web resources.
http://rattler.cameron.edu/prostate/

Internet Search

Search NIH WEB-SPACE
Search the National Institute of Medicines online database.
http://search.info.nih.gov

Search the NIH Guide Database
http://www.med.nyu.edu/keyword.html

National Library of Medicine
Search service to access the 9 million citations in MEDLINE, with links to participating online journals and other related databases.
http://www.ncbi.nlm.nih.gov/PubMed

Cancer News on the Net®
General resource with general cancer coverage including searching the Internet, cancer support groups and cancer book links.
http://www.cancernews.com/quickload.htm

General Internet Information

National Institutes of Health Home Page
A selection of some NIH health resources such as CancerNet, Clinical Alerts, the Women's Health Initiative, and the NIH Information Index (a subject-word guide to diseases and conditions under investigation at NIH).
http://www.nih.gov/ index.html

Yahoo!—Health Medicine
A Net-search resource for health and medical topics.
http://www.yahoo.com/health/medicine

An Introduction to Skin Cancer and Related Topics
http://www.maui.net/~southsky/introto.html

Journal of the American Medical Association
Peer-reviewed studies in clinical science, disease prevention, and health policy.
http://www.ama-assn.org/public/journals/jama

Human Health and Global Environmental Change
Consortium for International Earth Science Information Network, provides a human health bibliography.
http://www.ciesin.org/TG/HH/HH-ref.html

CancerGuide
http://cancerguide.org

Healthwise (Columbia University)
http://www.alice.columbia.edu

OncoLink Help Page (University of Pennsylvania)
http://oncolink.upenn.edu/about_oncolink/help.html

University of California at Berkeley Wellness Letter
http://www.enews.com/magazines/ucbwl

CNN Food and Health News Main Page
http://www.cnn.com/HEALTH/index.html

Your Health Daily
A New York Times syndicate of health-related articles.
http://nytsyn.com/med

CancerNet Web
CancerNet is a quick way to obtain cancer information from the National Cancer Institute (NCI). CancerNet lets you request information statements from the NCI's Physician Data Query database, fact sheets on various cancer topics from the NCI's Office of Cancer Communications.
http://www.ncc.go.jp/cnet.html

Food and Drug Administration Home Page
http://www.fda.gov

Combined Health Information Database
A combined database by the Department of Health and Human Services; the Public Health Service; the Centers for Disease Control and Prevention; and the National Institutes of Health.
http://chid.nih.gov

Centers for Disease Control and Prevention
http://www.cdc.gov

Internet Information on Food

International Food Information Council
Food safety and nutrition information.
http://ificinfo.health.org

The Vegetarian Society UK
http://www.vegsoc.org

The Vegetarian Society UK: Research Round-Up
http://www.veg.org/veg/Orgs/VegSocUK/Research/roundup1.html

Cooking, Food, and Nutrition
http://envirolink.org

Human Health and Nutrition
http://envirolink.org

Nutrition Advocate
http://envirolink.org/arrs/advocate/nut1.htm

The Vegetarian Resource Group (Home Page)
This link has vegetarian and vegan recipes, nutrition information, and journal excerpts.
http://www.vrg.org
http://envirolink.org

Other Resources

The National Center for Nutrition and Dietetics
A consumer hotline with recorded nutrition information and referrals for registered dietitians. (9:00 am to 4:00 pm central time, Monday through Friday) Messages available in Spanish.
(800) 366-1655

Center for Science in the Public Interest/Americans for Safe Food
1501 16th Street, NW
Washington, DC 20036
(202) 332-9110
http://www.cspinet.org/

Centers for Disease Control
Lead Poisoning and Prevention Branch
1600 Clifton Rd. NE
Atlanta, GA 30333

Centers for Disease Control
Division of Environmental Health Hazards and Health Effects
1600 Clifton Rd. NE
Atlanta, GA 30333

U.S. Environmental Protection Agency (EPA)
Office of Toxic Substances
401 M St., SW
Mail Code: TS 792, Room E539
Washington, DC 20460
EPA's Safe Drinking Water Hotline (800) 426-4791
EPA's RCRA Hotline (hazardous waste facilities) (800) 424-9346
EPA's Pollution Prevention Clearinghouse (202) 260-1023
EPA's Toxic Release Inventory (800) 535-0202
EPA's National Pesticide Telecommunications Network (800) 858-7378

Environmental Defense Fund
1616 P St. NW
Washington, DC 20036

Environmental Research Foundation
PO Box 5036
Annapolis, MD 21403
(410) 263-1584
E-mail: erf@rachel.clark.net
http://www.monitor.net/rachel/rehw-index.html

National Institute of Environmental Health
(919) 541-3345

Natural Resources Defense Council
http://www.11.nrdc.org

The Clearinghouse on Environmental Health Effects
(800) 643-4794

National Institute of Occupational Safety and Health
(800) 35-NIOSH

Occupational Safety and Health Administration
(800) 321-OSHA

National Center for Food and Agricultural Policy
1616 P Street NW
Washington, DC 20036
(202) 328-5048

U.S. Consumer Products Safety Commission
(301) 504-0580

Alliance to End Childhood Lead Poisoning
600 Pennsylvania Avenue, SE
Suite 1600
Washington, DC 20003

U.S. Food and Drug Administration
(202) 205-4943

For Further Reading

Introduction

Beardsley, T. A war not won: trends in cancer epidemiology. *Scientific Ameri* 270 (January 1994), 130–138.

Gloeckler Ries, L. A., et al. Cancer Statistics Review 1973–1989 [National Institutes of Health Publication No. 92-2789] Bethesda, MD: National Cancer Institute, 1992, Table I-3, pg. I.23.

Greig N. H. et al. Increasing annual incidence of primary malignant brain tumors in the elderly. *J Natl Cancer Inst* 82, no. 20 (October 17, 1990), pgs. 1621–24.

Hoel, D.G., et al. Trends in cancer mortality in 15 industrialized countries. *J Natl Cancer Inst* 84, no. 5 (March 4, 1992), 313–320.

Mao, Y., et al. Increasing brain cancer rates in Canada. *Canadian Med Assoc* 145, no. 12 (December 15, 1991), 1583–1591.

Chapter 1

Birt, D. F. and E. Bresnick, Chemoprevention by nonnutrient components of vegetables and fruits. In: *Cancer and Nutrition* (RB Alfin-Slater, and E. Kritchevsky, eds.) New York, Plenum Press, 1991; 221–60.

Couet, C., et al. Lactose and cataract in humans: A review. *J Am Coll Nutr* (1991) 10:79–86.

Cramer, D. W. and B. L. Harlow, Commentary: "A case-control study of milk drinking and ovarian cancer risk." *Am J Epidemiol* (1991) 134:454–56.

Drash, A. L., et al. Work group on cow's milk protein and diabetes mellitus. *Pediatrics* (1994) 94:752–54.

Friberg, L., et al. Cadmium and health: A toxicological and epidemiological appraisal. General aspects. Effects and response 1 and 2. Boca Raton, CRC Press, 1986.

Klassen, C. D., and J. B. Watkins, Mechanisms of bile formation, hepatic uptake, and biliary excretion. *Pharmacol Rev* (1984) 36:1–67.

Montgomery, R. K., et al. Lactose intolerance and the genetic regulation of intestinal-phlorizin hydrolase. *FASEB J.* (1991) 5:2824–32.

Rowland, I. R., et al. The effect of various dietary fibers on tissue concentration and chemical form of mercury after methylmercury exposure in mice. *Arch Toxicol* (1986) 59:94.

Segall, J. J. Dietary lactose as a possible risk factor for ischaemic heart disease: review of epidemiology. *Intern J Cardiol* (1994) 46:197–207.

Singal, R., et al. Glutathione: A first line of defense against cadmium toxicity. *FASEB J.* (1987) 1:220.

Snowdon, D. A. Animal product consumption and mortality because of all cancers combined, coronary heart disease, stroke, diabetes, and cancer in Seventh-Day Adventists. *Am J Clin Nutr* (1988) 48:739–748.

Story, J. A. and D. Kritchevsky. Comparison of the binding of bile acids and bile salts in vitro to several types of fiber. *J Nutr* (1976) 106:1292–94.

WHO IPCS Environmental Health Criteria 134. Cadmium. Geneva, World Health Organization, 1992.

Chapter 2

Blaylock, R. L., *Excitotoxins: The Taste That Kills*. Health Press, PO Drawer 1388, Santa Fe, NM 87504 1994.

Clark, W. R., *At War Within; The Double-Edged Sword of Immunity*. New York: Oxford University Press, 1995.

Fain, J. A. National trends in diabetes. An epidemiologic perspective. *Nursing Clinics of North America* (1993) 28:1–7.

Flegal, R. and D. R. Smith. Lead levels in preindustrial humans. *New Engl J Med* (1992) 326:1293–94.

Hoffman, C, et al., Persons with chronic conditions. *Ameri Med Assoc* 276, no. 18 (November 13, 1996), 1473–79.

Jacobson, J. L. and S. W. Jacobson, Dose-response in perinatal exposure to polychlorinated biphenyls (PCBs): the Michigan and North Carolina cohort studies. *Toxicol and Indust Health* 12, nos 3/4 (1996), 435–45.

Jacobson, J. L. and S. W. Jacobson, Intellectual impairment in children exposed to polychlorinated biphenyls in utero. *New Engl J Med* 335 no. 11 (September 12, 1996), 783–89.

Jernigan, D. B., et al., Minimizing the impact of drug-resistant streptococcus pneumonia (DRSP). *Ameri Med Assoc* (January 17, 1996), 206–9.

Kannan, K., et al. Elevated accumulation of tributyltin and its breakdown products in bottlenose dolphins (*Tursiops truncatus*) found stranded along the U.S. Atlantic and gulf coasts. *Environ Sci & Tech* 31, no. 1 (1997), 296–301.

Knox, E. G. Spatial clustering of childhood cancers in Great Britain. *J Epidem and Comm Health* 50, no. 3 (June 1996), 313–19.

Knox, E. G., and E. A. Gilman, Hazard proximities of childhood cancers in Great Britain from 1953–80. *J Epidem and Comm Health* 51 (1997), 151–59.

National Research Council (Bruce A. Fowler, editor), *Measuring Lead Exposure in Infants, Children, and Other Sensitive Populations.* Washington, DC: National Academy Press, 1993.

Olney, J. W., et al. Increasing brain tumor rates: is there a link to aspartame? *J of Neuropathology and Experimental Neurology* (1996) 55:1115–1123.

Raloff, J. Something's fishy, *Science News* (1994) 146:9.

Roberts, H. J. Does Aspartame Cause Human Brain Cancer? *Advancement in Medicine* (1991) 4:231–241.

Seachrist, L, Infections making a deadly comeback. *Science News* (1996) 149:38.

Statement of the work session on chemically-induced alterations in the developing immune system: the wildlife/human connection. *Environ Health Persp* (1996) 104:807–808.

Tilson, H. A., et al. Polychlorinated biphenyls and the developing nervous system: Cross-species comparisons. *Neurotoxicology and Teratology* (1990) 12:239–248.

Chapters 3 and 4

Chocolate: As hearty as red wine. *Science News* (1996) 150:235.

Demrow, H. S. et al. Administration of wine and grape juice inhibits in vivo platelet activity and thrombosis in stenosed canine coronary arteries. *Circulation* 1995 91:1182.

Milner, J. A. Reducing the risk of cancer. In: *Functional Foods*. New York: Van Nostrand Reinhold (1994), 39–70.

Stavric, B. Role of chemopreventers in human diet. *Clin Biochem* (1994) 27:319–332.

Waterhouse, A. L., et al. Antioxidants in chocolate. *Lancet* (1996) 348:834.

Watkins, T. R. Wine: Nutritional and Therapeutic Benefits. ACS Symposium Series 661, American Chemical Society, Washington, DC, 1997.

Chapter 5

Crowell, P. L. and M. N. Gould. Chemoprevention and therapy of cancer by d-limonene. *Crit Rev Oncogen* (1994) 5:1–22.

Gao, Y. T., et al. Reduced risk of esophageal cancer associated with green tea consumption. *J Natl Cancer Inst* (1994) 86:855–858.

Guengerich, F. P. and Kim, D. H. In vitro inhibition of dihydropyridine oxidation and aflatoxin B 1 activation in human liver microsomes by naringenin and other flavonoids. *Carcinogenesis* (1990) 11:2275–79

Kennedy, A. R. The evidence for soybean products as cancer preventive agents. *J Nutr* (1995) 125:733S–743S.

Komori, A., et al. Anticarcinogenic activity of green tea polyphenols. *Jpn J Clin Oncol* (1993) 23:186–190.

La Vecchia, C., et al. Tea consumption and cancer risk. *Nutr Cancer*, (1992) 17:27–31.

Mukhtar, H., et al. Green tea and skin-anticarcinogenic effects. *J Invest Derm* (1994) 102:3–7.

Yang, C. S., et al. Inhibition of tumorigenesis by chemicals from garlic and tea. *Adv Exp Med Biol* (1994) 354:113–22.

Yang, C. S. and Z. Y. Wang. Tea and cancer. *J Natl Cancer Inst* (1993) 85:1038–1049.

You, W. C. et al. Allium vegetables and reduced risk of stomach cancer. *J Natl Cancer Inst* 1989:81:162–164.

Chapter 6

Caragay, A. B. Cancer-preventive foods and ingredients. *Food Technology* (1992) 4665–68.

Gerhardsson de Verdier, M., et al. Meat, cooking methods and colorectal cancer: a case-referent study in Stockholm. *Int J Cancer* (1991) 49:1–6.

Gross, G. A., et al. Heterocyclic aromatic amine formation in grilled bacon, beef and fish in grill scrapings. *Carcinogenesis* (1993) 14:2313–18.

Hatch, F. T., et al. Quantitative correlation of mutagenic and carcinogenic potencies for heterocyclic amines from cooked foods and additional aromatic amines. *Mutat Res* (1992) 271:269–287.

Messina, M. The role of soy products in reducing risk of cancer. *J Natl Cancer Inst* (1991) 83(8):541–46.

Munro, I. C., et al. Safety assessment of ingested heterocyclic amines: Initial report. *Regul Toxicol Pharmacol* (1993) 17:S1.

Schwartz J. L. Beta carotene and/or vitamin E as modulators of alkylating agents in SCC-25 human squamous carcinoma cells. *Cancer Chemotherapy and Pharmacology* (1992) 29(3):207–13.

Steinmetz, K. A. Vegetables, fruit and cancer. I, Epidemiology. *Cancer Causes Control* (1991) 2(5):323–37.

Steinmetz, K. A. Vegetables, fruit, and cancer. II. Mechanisms. *Cancer Causes Control* (1991) 2(6):427–42.

Sugimura, T., et al. Heterocyclic amines in cooked food. In: *Food Toxicology A Perspective on the Relative Risk*. S. L. Taylor, R.A. Scanlan eds. New York: Marcel Dekker, 1989, 31–55.

Wattenberg, L. W. Inhibition of carcinogenesis by minor a nutrient constituents of the diet. *Proceedings of the Nutrition Society* (1990). 49(2):173–83.

Willet, W. C., et al. Intake of trans fatty acids and risk of coronary heart disease among women. *Lancet* (1993) 341:581–85.

Zhang, Y. A major inducer of anticarcinogenic protective enzymes from broccoli: isolation and elucidation of structure. *Proceedings of the National Academy of Sciences* (1992) 89:2399–2403.

Chapter 7

Bailey, L. B. (ed.) *Folate in Health and Disease.* New York: Marcel Dekker, 1994.

Bendich, A., and Butterworth, C. E. (eds.) *Micronutrients in Health and in Disease Prevention.* New York: Marcel Dekker, 1991.

Brag, G. and Ryan, D. (eds) Pennington Center Nutritional Series 3: Vitamins and Cancer Prevention. Louisiana: Baton Rouge University Press, 1993.

Cadenas, F., and Packer, L. (eds.) *Handbook of Antioxidants.* New York: Marcel Dekker, 1996.

Canfield, L. M., Krinsky, N. I., and Olson, J. A. (eds.) Carotenoids in Human Health 691. New York: *Annals of the New York Academy of Sciences,* 1993.

Henson, D. E. Ascorbic acid: Biologic functions and relation to cancer. *J Natl Cancer Inst* (1991), 83(8):547–550

Laidlaw, S. and Swendseid, H. (eds.) *Vitamins and Cancer Prevention: Contemporary Issues in Clinical Nutrition* 14. New York: J. Wiley and Sons, 1991.

Packer, L., and Fuchs, J. (eds.) *Vitamin E in Health and Disease.* New York: Marcel Dekker, 1993.

Picciano, M. F., Stokstadt, F. L. R., and Gregory, J. F. (eds.) *Folic Acid Metabolism in Health and Disease: Contemporary Issues in Clinical Nutrition* 13. New York: Wiley Liss, 1990.

Chapter 8

Adlecreutz, H. Diet and breast cancer. *Acta Oncalogica.* (1992) 31(2):175–81.

Apter, D. Hormonal events during female puberty in relation to breast cancer risk. *Eur J Cancer Prev* 5, no. 6 (1996), 476–82.

Barnes, S. Soybeans inhibit mammary tumors in models of breast cancer. *Progress in Clinical and Biological Research.* (1990) 347:239–53.

Bresnick, E. Reduction in mammary tumorigenesis in the rat by cabbage and cabbage residue. *Carcinogenesis* (1990) 11(7):1159–63.

Davis D. L. and Bradlow, H. L. Can environmental estrogens cause breast cancer? *Scientific Ameri* 273, no. 4 (October, 1995) 166–72.

Davis, D. L., et al. Medical hypothesis: Xenoestrogens as preventable causes of breast cancer. *Envir Health Persp* 101 (October 1993), 372–77.

Herman-Giddens, M. E. et al. Secondary sexual characteristics and menses in young girls seen in office practice: a study from the pediatric research in office settings network. *Pediatrics* 99, no. 4 (April 1997), 505–512.

Holm, L. E. Treatment failure and dietary habits in women with breast cancer. *J Natl Cancer Inst* (1993) 85(1):32–36.

Howe, G. E. Dietary factors and risk of breast cancer: combined analysis of 12 case-control studies. *J Natl Cancer Inst* (1990) 82(7):561–69.

Jellinck, P. H., et al. Influence of indole-3-carbinol on the hepatic microsomal formation of catechol estrogens. *Steroids* (1991) 56:446–450.

MacKenzie, I. Breast cancer following multiple fluoroscopies. *Brit J Cancer* 19 (1965), 1–8.

Marshall, E. Search for a Killer: focus shifts from fat to hormones. *Science* (1993) 259:618–21.

Michnovicz, J. J. and H. L. Bradlow. Altered estrogen metabolism and excretion in humans following consumption of indole-3-carbinol. *Nutr Cancer* (1991) 16:59–66.

Rose, D. P. High-fiber diet reduces serum estrogen concentrations in premenopausal women. *Ameri J Clin Nutr* (1991) 54(3):520–25.

Sternberg, S. Aspirin users may trim breast cancer risk. *Science News* 149 (February 24, 1996), 116.

Stoll, B. A., et al. Does early physical maturity influence breast cancer risk? *Acta Oncologica*, 33, no. 2 (1994), 171–76.

Tiwari, R, K, et al. Selective responsiveness of human breast cancer cells to indole-3-carbinol, a chemopreventive agent. *J Natl Cancer Inst* (1994) 86:126–131.

Tiwary, C. M, Premature sexual development in children following the use of placenta and/or estrogen containing hair product(s). *Ped Research* 135 (1994), 108A. Abstract.

Wanebo, C. K., et al. Breast cancer after exposure to the atomic bombings of Hiroshima and Nagasaki. *New Engl J Med* 279 (1968), 667–71.

Wolff, M. S., et al. Blood levels of organochlorine residues and risk of breast cancer. *J Natl Cancer Inst* 85 (April 21, 1993), 648–52.

Chapter 9

Bower, B. Excess lead linked to boys' delinquency. *Science News*, 149 (February 10, 1996), 86.

Jacobson, J. L. and S. W. Jacobson. Intellectual impairment in children exposed to polychlorinated biphenyls in utero. *New Engl J Med*, 335 no. 11 (September12, 1996), 783–89.

Mahaffery, K. R. Nutritional factors in lead poisoning. *Nutr Rev* (1981) 39:353.

Moffitt, T. E. Measuring children's antisocial behaviors. *J Ameri Med Assoc* 275, no. 5 (February 7, 1996), 403–4.

Needleman, H. L., et al. Bone lead levels and delinquent behavior, *J Ameri Med Assoc* 275, no. 5 (February 7, 1996), 363–69.

NRC. *Measuring Lead Exposure in Infants, Children and Other Sensitive Populations.* Washington, DC: National Academy Press, 1993.

Chapter 10

Brawley, O. W., et al. 5 alpha reductase inhibition and prostate cancer prevention. *Cancer Epidemiol, Biomarkers, Prev* (1994) 3:177–82.

Chan, J. M., et al. Plasma insulin-like growth factor-I and prostate cancer risk: A prospective study. *Science* (1998) 279:563–66.

Checkoway, H., et al. Medical, lifestyle, and occupational risk factors for prostate cancer. *Prostate* (1987) 10:79–88.

Corder, E. H. Vitamin D and prostate cancer: A prediagnostic study with stored sera Cancer Epidemiol, Biomarkers, *Prev* (1993) 2:467–472.

Depue, R. H., et al. Estrogen exposure during gestation and risk of testicular cancer. *J Natl Cancer Inst* (1983) 71:1151–1155.

Giovannucci, E., et al. A prospective study of dietary fat and risk of prostate cancer. *J Natl Cancer Inst,* (1993) 85;1571–79.

Giovannucci, E., et al. Carotenoids and retinol in relation to risk of prostate cancer. *J Natl Cancer Inst* (1995) 87:1767–76.

Heshmat, M. Y., et al. Nutrition and prostate cancer. A case control study. *Prostate* (1985) 6:457–60.

Hirayama, T. Epidemiology of prostate cancer with special reference to the role of diet. *Natl Cancer Instr Mongr* (1979) 53: 149–55.

Kaul, L., et al. The role of diet in prostate cancer. *Nutr Cancer* (1987) 9: 123–128.

Kolonel, L. N., et al. Diet and prostate cancer: A case-control study in Hawaii. *Ameri J Epidemiol* (1988) 127: 999–1012.

LeMarchland, L., et al. Animal fat consumption and prostate cancer: A prospective study in Hawaii. *Epidemiol* (1994) 133:276–82.

Nakayama, O., et al. Riboflavin, a testosterone 5-alpha-reductase inhibitor. *J Antibiotics* (1990) 43:1615–1616.

Pinczowski, D., et al. Occurrence of testicular cancer in patients operated on for cryptorchism and inguinal hernia. *J Urol* (1991) 146:1291–1294.

Ragan, H. A and Mast, T. J. Cadmium inhalation and male reproductive toxicity. *Reviews of Environmental Contamination and Toxicology* 114 (1990), 1–22.

Ross, R. K., et al. Do diet and androgens alter prostate cancer risk via a common etiologic pathway? *J Natl Cancer Inst* (1994) 86:251–54.

Chapter 11

Anderson, R. Assessment of the roles of vitamin C, vitamin E, and B-carotene in the modulation of oxidant stress mediated by cigarette smoke-activated phagocytes. *Am J Clin Nutr* (1991) 53:358S–361S.

Freudenheim, J. L. Lifetime alcohol intake and risk of rectal cancer in western New York. *Nutrition and Cancer* (1990) 13:101–9.

Kaufman, D. W., et al. Tar content of cigarettes in relation to lung cancer. *Am J Epidemiol* (1989) 129:703–11.

Mezey, E, Metabolic effects of alcohol. *Fed. Proc,* (1985) 44:134–138.

Nagano, U., et al. High density lipoprotein loses its effect to stimulate efflux of cholesterol from foam cells after oxidative modification. *Proc Natl Acad Sci U.S.A.* (1991) 88:6457–61.

Naruszewica, M., et al. Oxidative modification of lipoprotein (a) and the effect of b-carotene. *Metabolism* (1992) 41:1215–24.

Schectman, G., et al. The influence of smoking or vitamin C status in adults. *Am J Public Health.* (1989) 79:158–162.

Schectman, K. and Moser, U. The influence of smoking on vitamin C status in adults. *Am J Public Health* (1989) 79:158–162.

Chapter 12

Alberts, D. S. Effects of dietary wheat bran fiber on rectal epithelial cell proliferation in patients with resection for colorectal cancers. *J Natl Cancer Inst* (1990) 82:1280–85.

Anti, M. Effect of omega-3 fatty adds on rectal mucosal cell proliferation in subjects at risk for colon cancer. *Gastroenterol* (1992) 103:883–91.

DeCosse, J. J. Effect of wheat fiber and vitamins C and E on rectal polyps in patients with familial adenomatous polyposis. *J Natl Cancer Inst* (1989) 81(17):1290–97.

Goodinan, M. T. Dietary factors in lung cancer prognosis. *Eur J Cancer* (1992) 28(2/3):495–501.

Howe, G. R. Dietary intake of fiber and decreased risk of cancers of the colon and rectum: evidence from the combined analysis of 13 case-control studies *J Natl Cancer Inst* (1992) 84(24):1887–96.

Willett, W. C. Relation of meat, fat, and fiber intake to the risk of colon cancer in a prospective study among women. *New Engl J Med* (1990) 323:1664–72.

Chapter 13

Ginsberg, P. *The Whole Soy Cookbook.* Random House, Inc. Westminster, MD 1998.

Messina, M., and Messina, V. *The Dietitian's Guide to Vegetarian Diets.* Gaithersburg, Maryland: Aspen Publishers, Inc. 1996).

Raichlen S. *High-Flavor, Low-fat Cooking.* New York: Penguin, 1994.

Raichlen S. *High-Flavor, Low-fat Vegetarian Cooking,* New York, Viking, 1995.

Glossary

Acetaldehyde
The primary conversion product of alcohol (ethanol) that occurs in the liver. It is known to exert toxic properties on the liver and other organ systems.

Acetaminophen
The active ingredient in a number of analgesics or pain killers. Acetaminophen is detoxified by glutathione. In larger doses causes toxicity to the liver and can make you more vulnerable to environmental chemicals and alcohol.

Aflatoxin
A family of mold toxins that are produced by the fungus Aspergillus flavus. Aflatoxins are some the most potent cancer-causing agents known. They occur as contaminates in food, particularly cereals and peanuts. Any crop that comes in contact with soil and is stored in warm and humid conditions can harbor aflatoxins.

Allium plants
A strong-smelling bulb plant of the lily family, such as garlic, onion, leeks, and shallots.

Alpha-5-reductase enzyme
A reducing enzyme that speeds the reaction of testosterone into 5 alpha-dihydrotestosterone (DHT). This is an irreversible conversion that takes place notably in the prostate gland.

Alzheimer's disease
A senile dementia that is usually seen in persons over 50 years. The brain has specific tissue changes that include evidence of extensive lipid peroxidation.

Amino acids
A large group of organic compounds that are the building blocks for making proteins.

Anabolic steroids
Anabolic steroids were developed in the 1930s as drugs to replace the sex hormone testosterone. There are twenty or more varieties that cause rapid gains in muscle mass and strength. Anabolic steroid use can increase the risk of future cancer of the prostate gland, testes, and liver.

Aneurysm
The splitting or tearing of the layers that make up the walls of the arteries. This weakens the vessel wall and is often accompanied with a large balloonlike swelling that can burst. Aneurysms can occur in the major artery leaving the heart (aortic aneurysms) or within the brain.

Antibacterial
Prevents, or is destructive to, the growth of bacteria.

Antibodies
A group of substances usually formed by the immune system. They are formed in the presence of antigens, or foreign agents like bacteria.

Anticancer
A substance that has been shown to prevent, block, or reverse the progression of cancer.

Antifeedants
A substance that is toxic to insects and inhibits the feeding activities. The citrus liminoids (limonene) are an example of antifeedants.

Antifungal
A compound that prevents or is antagonistic to the growth of mold, yeast, or fungi.

Anti-inflammatory
A drug or agent that blocks or lessens an inflammatory reaction.

Antimitotic
A substance that impedes cell cycling or cell division.

Antimutagenic
A compound that blocks or prevents DNA or other nucleic acids from sustaining a permanent chemical change.

Antioxidant
An agent that inhibits oxidation, as in preventing the rancidity of fats and oils or the deterioration of other materials.

Antioxidant enzymes
A series of enzymes that detoxify activated species of oxygen, such as superoxide anion and hydrogen peroxide.

Antithrombotic
A substance that, usually by modifying the platelet response, prevents or lessens the chance of forming a clot or thrombus.

Antitumor
A compound that hinders the growth and survival of tumors.

Antiviral
An agent that abolishes or weakens the action of a virus.

Aplastic anemia
A condition characterized by defective regeneration of red blood cells. It involves an injury to the stem cells that mature into red blood cells.

Arachidonic acid
An unsaturated fat that is essential in nutrition and is converted into prostaglandins. It is a central chemical involved in inflammatory reactions and formation of other active agents. Meat is a rich dietary source of arachidonic acid. Aspirin and other anti-inflammatory agents work by blocking the conversion of arachidonic acid into certain active prostaglandin products. This may be the central reason aspirin protects from heart attacks.

Arsenic
A metalloid used in agricultural products and the manufacture of glass and metals. Arsenic is easily absorbed from breathing or ingestion and it accumulates in hair, skin, and nails.

Asbestos
The name given to two general families of fibrous minerals: chrysotile and amphiboles. Asbestos dust can be toxic to the lung from breathing. It can cause a loss of lung function and lung cancer, especially in smokers.

Ascorbic acid
A vitamin present in citrus fruits, green vegetables, and tomatoes that is necessary for the proper assembly of collagen. It also has many anticancer properties and blocks the formation of nitrosamines.

Aspergillus flavus
A mold fungus that can produce a series of chemicals called aflatoxins.

Asthma
A disease that is characterized by an exaggerated response of the airways to restrict and narrow to the point where the person has difficulty breathing.

Atherosclerosis
A disease condition associated with excessive connective tissue, resulting in a thickening of the inner surface of blood vessels. This results in loss of flexibility (elasticity) and a narrowing or constriction of arteries. Atherosclerosis increases the risk for a heart attack and stroke.

234 EAT TO BEAT CANCER

Attention deficit disorder (ADD)
A disorder found in children, characterized by a short attention span, poor memory, and an inability to follow directions. Lead exposure has been shown to cause ADD.

Autoimmune disease
A disease that results in an immune reaction directed against your own DNA, RNA, or other normal cell components. Systemic lupus erythematosus is a common autoimmune disease.

Basal cell carcinoma
A cancer or tumor that is derived from the deepest layer of the epidermis (basal cells) in the skin. In humans this form of skin cancer is well contained and benign. It may infiltrate other tissues if not removed by surgery.

Benign prostatic hypertrophy
A nonmalignant condition in which the prostate gland grows in size.

Benzene
A clear, inflammable aromatic liquid that is used as a solvent for making dyes, lacquers, and varnishes; also used as an octane-booster for gasoline. It is generally agreed to cause leukemia.

Benzo[a]pyrene (BAP)
A cancer-producing chemical from the family of polycyclic aromatic hydrocarbons. BAP is formed as a byproduct in many combustion and incineration processes. It is found in cigarette smoke, air pollution, and processed or charbroiled food.

Beta carotene
A class of carotenoid that is widely distributed and part of a large family of over 600 yellow, orange, and red plant pigments, notably in carrots. Beta carotene is converted into vitamin A.

Bile
A green fluid secreted by the gall bladder into the small intestine. Bile acts like a soap, breaking fat into a mixture that can be absorbed into the blood. Primary bile acids can be converted by bacteria that reside in the intestine into secondary bile acids. Secondary bile acids are more toxic to the surfaces of the large intestine.

Biliary secretion
The process of bile formation in the liver and storage in the gall bladder, and finally secretion into the small intestine. Pronounced secretion of bile occurs after eating high fat meals.

Bilirubin
A yellow-colored breakdown product from hemoglobin that does not contain iron and is excreted in the bile. If bilirubin is not properly excreted in bile it can build up in tissues, causing a yellow discoloration (jaundice).

Biotin
A member of the B vitamins, B2 group, found in egg yolk and yeast.

Blood brain barrier
A specialized barrier in the capillaries of the brain and spinal cord. It prevents the entry of many chemicals that easily cross into other organs.

Cadmium
A metal used in batteries, electroplating, paint pigments, and as a stabilizer for plastics. Cadmium is toxic to the kidney and liver, and is linked to prostate cancer.

Canavanine
An amino acid analog that is very similar in structure to the amino acid arginine.

Cancer
A general term that refers to upwards of 300 different, uncontrolled growths or neoplasms, that invade surrounding tissues and may eventually cause death to the host.

Canthaxanthin
A carotenoid that is widely distributed and part of a large family of over 600 yellow, orange, and red plant pigments.

Carbon disulfide
An industrial chemical used in the manufacture of rubber. It is well known to cause toxicity to the nervous system.

Carcinogen
Any agent or substance that causes cancer.

Cardiomyopathy
Collectively a series of disease changes that result in abnormal functions of the heart muscle.

Cataract
A loss of transparency in the lens of the eye.

Catechin
A plant chemical from the tannin group. Green tea is a rich source of catechins.

Cell membrane
A fat or lipid bi-layer that forms the outer structural basis of cells.

Chelated minerals
A chemical group that is bonded to a metal ion facilitating its uptake or transport.

Chemoprevention
The science of substances known to suppress or prevent cancer. It uses whole fresh foods and food chemicals and drugs to prevent, stop, and even reverse the progression of cancer.

Chemotherapy
Treatment of cancer with toxic chemical agents. Chemotherapeutic agents often work by blocking the cell division of the tumor. They also are toxic to, and block, normal cell division. Consequently they have a number of severe side effects, such as nausea and vomiting, loss of hair, intestinal disturbances, irreversible kidney damage, and hearing loss.

Chlorophyll
Green plant pigments that absorb UV wavelengths of light and donate electrons for the process of photosynthesis.

Cholesterol
The most abundant steroid present in animal tissue, especially in the brain, animal fat, egg yolk, and bile. It is normally transported in the blood and is a main component of gallstones.

Choline
It is part of the vitamin B complex and is essential for making certain amino acids.

Chromosomes
The microscopic rod-shaped bodies that are contained in the nucleus of the cell. They contain the genes and transmit the hereditary characteristics of the individual.

Chronic Fatigue Syndrome (CFS)
A syndrome in which the person becomes severely fatigued. It usually hits after an infection like mononucleosis or Epstein-Barr virus. CFS does not have an effective treatment.

Chronic illness
Denotes an illness that slowly progresses and continues for a long duration and usually is resistant to treatment.

Cleft palate
A birth defect resulting from the incomplete merging of the embryonic processes that form the roof of the mouth, palate, or upper lips.

Clostridia botulinum
The causative bacteria in a form of food poisoning called botulism.

Cofactor
A vitamin, group, or ion such as magnesium, essential for enzyme action.

Colloidal
Molecules or aggregates that, when dispersed in a solvent, remain uniformly suspended and do not form a true solution.

Complex carbohydrate
A sugar molecule that is highly complex. Complex carbohydrates take longer to process and are usually present in high-fiber foods.

Computed Axial Tomography (CAT)
A computer-constructed imaging technique that reconstructs thin slices of tissue from X-ray data.

Contact inhibition
A process that triggers cell division to turn off. This process is lost when cells turn cancerous.

Coronary heart disease (CHD)
Generic description for three forms of heart disease: arteriosclerotic heart disease, a physical narrowing of the arteries that feed that heart; myocardial infarction, a catastrophic form of CHD from a sudden blockage of coronary arteries that damages the heart muscle; angina pectoris, a condition that results in severe chest pains from inadequate blood flow to the heart.

Cruciferous vegetables
A family of plants with the arrangement of petals in the shape of a cross, as in cabbage, broccoli, and watercress. They have potent anticancer properties.

Cyanide
An extremely toxic substance that has the odor of bitter almonds.

DDT
Abbreviation for dichlorodiphenyltrichloroethane. A chlorinated pesticide that was widely used to control insects, especially mosquitoes. Although banned in the 1970s, it persists in the environment.

DES (diethylstilbestrol)
A synthetic, orally active compound with more potent estrogen activity than naturally produced estrogen.

DHEA (dehydro-3-epiandrosterone)
A steroid hormone produced primarily in the adrenal glands.

Dilantin
A drug used to control seizures in conditions like epilepsy.

Dioxin
A toxic chemical contaminate in the herbicide Agent Orange.

DNA
The abbreviation for deoxyribonucleic acid, DNA is an essential component of all living matter. The basic material in the chromosomes that include the genetic code and transmit the hereditary characteristics.

DNA repair enzymes
A collection of enzymes that scan DNA for deletions and errors.

Dose response
A relationship between the administered dose and the extent of toxicity or toxic injury produced by a chemical or drug.

Ectopic pregnancy
A pregnancy that occurs outside the cavity of the uterus. It does not develop normally and sometimes has to be surgically removed.

Electrons
A negatively charged unit of matter that orbits around the atomic nucleus (proton).

Ellagic acid
A natural plant chemical found in a variety of fruits and vegetables.

Emphysema
A disease characterized by a loss of lung function. This can result from either a loss of alveolar sacs where oxygen exchange occurs, or it can affect the bronchioles.

Endometriosis
A disease of the endometrial tissue of the uterus, frequently involving cysts.

Endoscopy
The visual examination of the interior of a canal or hollow structure with an instrument called the endoscope.

Enteric-coated (aspirin)
A special coating on pills that hinders the release of the drug in the stomach. This is especially useful in reducing the toxicity that aspirin exerts to the lining of the stomach.

Enterolactone
Produced in the human body from plant chemicals or lignans. Rich sources of lignans include soy and flaxseed.

Enzyme
A protein that speeds up or catalyzes chemical reactions in other substances but remains unchanged in the chemical process.

Epithelia
The purely cellular layer covering all free surfaces that lacks blood vessels, as in mucous membranes or lining the ducts of the breast.

Epstein-Barr virus
A herpes virus that was first described in 1964 by Epstein and Barr.

Essential fats
The human body can make all of the fats it needs from carbohydrates except two: linoleic acid and linolenic acid. Since they must be supplied in the diet, they are termed essential. The essential fats are widely distributed in plant and seed oils.

Estrogen
Female sex hormone. Higher levels of estrogen have been linked to breast cancer.

Fibrocystic breast disease
A condition of cyst growth within the fibrous connective tissue of the breast.

Flavonoids
A group of over 4,000 naturally occurring plant compounds, also called bioflavonoids and polyphenols. They are widely distributed in fruits and vegetables.

Foam cells
Abnormal white blood cells that form as a result of oxidized fats or fried food.

Folic acid (folacin, foleate)
A vitamin that is critical to the making of all new cells. Folic acid is used together with vitamin B12 to manufacture DNA.

Follicle
A cellular mass containing an egg in the ovary.

Formaldehyde
A highly reactive chemical that is irritating to the upper respiratory tract and causes cancerous growths in exposed rats. It is widely used in industry and is a component of carpet adhesives, particle boards, and foam insulation.

Free radical
A chemical species with an unpaired electron in the outer shell. Normally electrons are paired for stability, as the free (unpaired) electron makes the chemical unstable and reactive.

Free range
Poultry or beef that is raised and allowed to graze unrestricted in a free range environment. This is in stark contrast to the factory style feed lots that crowd animals into stalls and use extensive antibiotics and growth stimulants.

Fungi
A large group of simple plants that lack chlorophyll, as in mold, mildews, yeast, and mushrooms.

Fungicide
An agent that inhibits or kills the growth of fungi.

Gastrointestinal system
Relating to the stomach and intestines.

Germ tissue
The embryo of a seed, as in wheat germ.

Glial cells
Branched, connective tissue that binds and supports the nervous tissue.

Glioma
A tumor or cancerous growth that arises in glial cells.

Glucosinates
Over 100 biologically active substances found in cruciferous vegetables.

Glutathione
A powerful cellular antioxidant involved in detoxification.

Glutathione-S-transferase (GST)
A detoxifying liver enzyme that can speed up and assist in the removal of pollutants from the body.

Glycrrhiza (licorice root)
The dried root of Glycyrrhiza radix and other species.

Hepatitis
Hepatitis A, B, and C commonly cause liver disease. Type A is most commonly acquired from contaminated food and water. Type B is often sexually transmitted and obtained by the use of contaminated hypodermic needles. Type C causes chronic liver disease, is linked to liver cancer, and is transmitted sexually or through contaminated needles.

Hepatocellular carcinoma
A cancerous growth or tumor that arises from the liver cells.

Heterocyclic amines (HAs)
A series of over twenty complex chemicals that are formed during high-temperature cooking. HAs are formed in high-protein foods, especially red meat.

Hodgkin's disease
A malignant cancer that involves a white cell disorder, characterized by an enlargement of the lymph nodes. It commonly afflicts adolescent and young adult males.

Homocysteine
An amino acid that is converted into methionine. Homocysteine levels build up when the diet is poor in vitamins B6, B12, and folic acid. Homocysteine has been found to promote heart disease.

Human papilloma viruses
A virus family of over sixty different members that have been isolated from malignant and benign growths. They are linked to cervical cancer.

Hydralzine
A drug that is used to treat high blood pressure on a long-term basis.

Immune system
A complex assembly of antibodies and specialized white blood cells that protect the body from foreign agents such as bacteria.

Indole-3-carbinol
A natural constituent of cruciferous vegetables that blocks the growth of tumors.

Initiation
Considered the first phase in the progression of cancer, where cells are exposed to a cancer-producing agent. During this stage an irreversible change takes place in the DNA of initiated cells that make it more sensitive to other chemical exposures.

Insulin
A protein hormone made by the beta cells of pancreatic islets. Insulin lowers the blood sugar levels and influences fat and amino acid conversions.

Intraductal carcinoma
A cancer that arises within the duct system of the breast but has not invaded the adjacent breast tissue.

Isoflavones
A subset of flavonoids that are found mostly in legumes like soybeans.

Isoniazid
A drug used to treat tuberculosis.

Leukocytes
A white blood cell that plays an important role in the body's defense against infection.

Lignan
Chemical building blocks for lignin, a major component that strengthens cell walls of plants. Soy, and especially flax seeds, are a rich source of dietary plant lignans.

Limonene
Limonene is a potent anticancer compound that is found in citrus oils, caraway, thyme, cardamom, and orange flower.

Lipid peroxidation
Free radicals in the presence of lipids are capable of extracting hydrogen atoms from the lipid (fat), thereby generating a free radical. The lipid becomes unstable and oxygen may react with it, degrading its structure.

Lipoproteins
Compounds that ferry lipids through the blood to tissue sites. They consist of blood protein and fat.

Lobular carcinoma
An invasive form of breast cancer that accounts for about 10 percent of the total cancer.

Lou Gehrig's disease
A progressive and usually fatal neuromuscular disease.

Lymph
A clear yellowish fluid (lympha) containing various white blood cells that is found in intercellular spaces and flows in specialized lymphatic vessels.

Macular degeneration
The most common disorder in the eye of the elderly that leads to blindness.

Magnetic resonance imaging (MRI)
An imaging technique first used to examine humans in the early 1980s. While more costly, a distinct advantage of MRI is that it does not use X-rays or other radiation like CAT scans.

Mammograms
A radio-imaging technique that is used to screen for breast cancer.

Manganese
An essential mineral.

Medullary carcinoma
An invasive cancer of the breast that involves about 5 to 10 percent of all breast cancer.

Melanin
One of the naturally occurring pigments located in the skin and retina. It protects the skin in response to UV light exposure.

Melanoma
A malignant tumor that is derived from the pigment cells in the skin.

Melatonin
A hormone formed in the pineal gland located in the brain. Melatonin is an antioxidant, which is secreted at night and induces sleep.

Mercury
A metallic element that is liquid at room temperature. Methyl mercury is the organic form that accumulates in fish and seafood from environmental contamination.

Methionine
An amino acid that contains sulfur and is important in the manufacture and repair of DNA.

Methyl groups
Methyl groups are critical components for the repair of DNA.

Mitochondria
A vesicle inside cells that liberates the energy stored in sugars and fats.

Monoterpenes
A phytochemical group that is found in citrus oils and spices like mint, caraway, thyme, coriander, and cardamom.

Monounsaturated fat
A fat (triglyceride) in which one or more fatty acids lack hydrogen atoms. Monounsaturated fats are linked to preventing heart disease. Examples include olive oil, canola oil, and macadamia nut oil.

Mucinous carcinoma
A rare form of breast cancer.

Multiple chemical sensitivity (MCS)
A newly described disease, also called environmental illness, that seems to affect the immune and nervous systems. The symptoms of MCS involve insomnia, dizziness, depression, mood swings, and a large collection of other symptoms. People with MCS show extreme sensitivity to very low levels of various chemicals including formaldehyde, perfumes, paint solvents, household cleaners, new building materials, tobacco smoke, and vehicle exhaust.

Multiple myeloma
A malignant disorder that involves the expansion of a single antibody. It is common in those who have suffered a prolonged infection such as pneumonia or tuberculosis.

Multiple sclerosis (MS)
A chronic disease that is characterized by speech defects, spastic movements, or a loss of muscular coordination. MS is common in countries where the population consumes high quantities of meat, dairy, and processed foods that are low in essential fats. In contrast, MS is rare in countries that consume high amounts of essential fats as in seed oils, olive oil, fish oils, and fresh fruits and vegetables.

Mutagen
A substance or agent that causes permanent changes in the DNA, or mutations. Ionizing radiation is a very potent mutagen.

Neoplasm
Literally a new growth, that grows without any form of coordination with the host.

Neural tube
A primitive tubular structure that is formed early in the embryo and matures into the brain and spinal cord. Folic acid is critical to its proper development.

Niacin
An essential nutrient that is found in nuts and grains. It is a critical factor in energy production.

Nitrates
Nitrates are found in normal diets in cured meats, vegetables such as spinach, beets, radishes, and some cheeses. Cured or salted and smoked meat is preserved with sodium nitrates. Nitrates are especially high in commercially grown produce that uses high-nitrogen fertilizers.

Nitrites
Nitrites are formed from nitrate by bacterial nitrate reductase that can be found in the oral cavity or within the GI tract.

Nitrosamines
Nitrosamines are powerful carcinogens that can be formed in the stomach from the presence of both nitrite and amino compounds.

Non-Hodgkin's lymphoma (NHL)
NHL are the other major forms of lymphoma that distinguish it from Hodgkin's disease. It is characterized by painless and progressive enlargement of lymphoid tissue such as lymph glands. The incidence is lowest in the developing nations and highest in the U.S.

Organochlorine chemicals
A series of fat-soluble compounds such as DDT, PCBs, and dioxin.

Organosulfurous compounds
A group of seventy or more compounds that are contained in allium plants.

Organotin compounds
A toxic metal complex that is used in agricultural pesticides, stabilizers for the plastic PVC, and as antifouling bottom paints for boats. They cause toxicity to the nervous system.

Osteoporosis
A progressive bone-thinning disease that usually afflicts women and some elderly men.

Oxidation
The combination with oxygen, or the process where electrons are removed from atoms or molecules.

Pap smear
A screening test for cancer of the cervix.

Parkinson's disease
A chronic disease of the nervous system that results in tremors, muscle rigidity, and an abnormal gait while walking.

Partially hydrogenated vegetable oil
This is a food-processing technique in which hydrogen is added to oils. It causes the formation of unnatural trans-fatty acids. Trans-fatty acids are not formed in the body and are rarely found in nature. The partially hydrogenated oils are more creamy and extend shelf life of food products. A healthful diet should avoid trans-fatty acids.

pH
A symbol for the degree of acidity or alkalinity in solution.

Phase II enzymes
A collection of enzymes involved in transforming chemicals from fat soluble into water soluble versions. This is a critical process of chemical removal that mostly takes place in the liver.

Phytochemicals
A large family of non-nutritive factors from plants that play the major role in preventing cancer.

Phytoestrogens
Plant compounds that compete with the activity of estrogen. Soy products are rich sources of phytoestrogens and are believed to protect from breast cancers and some others.

Platelets
Small rod-shaped corpuscles in the blood that are centrally involved in the blood-clotting process.

Polyamines
A group of bioactive substances that include: spermine, spermidine, putrescine, and cadaverine.

Polychlorinated biphenyls (PCBs)
A family of chemicals that have been used since the 1930s in electrical transformers. They damage the immune system.

Potassium
A metallic element that occurs in nature always in combination with other elements or compounds. It is critical to maintaining the heartbeat and is found in many vegetables and fruit.

Procainamide
A drug used to treat a variety of irregular heartbeats.

Promotion
Promotion is one of the stages of progression on the road to cancer. A variety of chemicals are termed promoters and have been shown to induce promotion; for instance, both estrogen and testosterone promote cancer. Other examples include the secondary bile acids (colon cancer), saccharin (bladder cancer), and phenobarbital (liver cancer). Promoters do not interfere with the DNA-like initiators, and the effects are reversible if the promoter is withdrawn before a cancer erupts.

Prostaglandins
A family of biologically active lipids (fats) that have widespread functions, as in platelet clumping, inflammation, hormone production, blood pressure, smooth muscle contraction, and gastric secretion.

Prostaglandins are very potent compounds also involved with cancer progression. Aspirin is known to block the production of certain prostaglandins.

Prostate gland
A male sex gland that produces a fluid that increases the pH of semen and activates the sperm.

Prostate-specific antigen (PSA)
A protein that is produced in greater levels in men who have prostate cancer or the condition called benign prostatic hyperplasia. Monitoring PSA levels is a method to determine the general growth rate of the cancer.

Protease inhibitor
A substance that blocks enzymes that are capable of breaking down proteins. Soybeans and many other seeds contain protease inhibitors.

Psyllium
Psyllium is the seed of the plantain plant. Both the seeds and their hulls are edible. The seeds have been used in Europe for intestinal health since the 16th century.

Quercetin
A series of flavonoid compounds that have potent anticancer properties. Sources for quercetin include fruits, vegetables (especially red onions), and cereal grains.

Radiation therapy
A cancer therapy that uses high-energy X-rays and gamma rays to damage the DNA of tumors and impede their growth. Radiation therapy is a routine procedure for many cancers treated in the early stages like breast cancer and Hodgkin's disease. Unfortunately it also causes widespread damage to adjacent healthy tissues, and thereby increases the risk of further cancer.

Radiolytic products
Sterilizing food by the action of X-rays or irradiation forms new products (radiolytic).

Radon
A radioactive gas that arises from the atomic disintegration of radium. Radon gas can enter homes through the flooring and cause toxicity and lung cancer.

Rash guard
A lightweight, water-repelling garment worn to prevent the skin from chaffing while wearing a wetsuit. Rash guards block sun exposure.

Reserpine
A plant extract that is used as a drug for controlling blood pressure.

Resveratrol
A compound found in grape skins and red wine that lessens heart disease and stroke.

Retinoid
A family of compounds similar to vitamin A.

Saponins
Plant chemicals commonly found in legumes and other plants that are associated with reducing tumor growth and abnormal growth of cells in the colon. They are similar in structure to cholesterol. Yet they have been found to bind cholesterol and reduce its absorption.

Scirrhous carcinoma
A cancer that arises in the ducts of the female breast. Scirrhous cancer is known by a stony hard tumor and accounts for over 75 percent of breast cancer. When all forms of ductal cancer are tallied, over 90 percent of breast cancer arises in the ductal epithelial cells.

Scrotum
In males a pouch of skin that externally contains the testicles.

Scurvy
A disease associated with deficiency of vitamin C.

Selenium
A metallic element associated with decreased risk of cancers.

Simple carbohydrates
Smaller-sized sugars, as in sucrose, that are often added in great amounts to processed food. High-sugar diets are a risk factor for heart disease.

Singlet oxygen
An activated form of oxygen that is more reactive and toxic. Beta carotene takes the punch out of the toxicity of singlet oxygen.

Skin cancer
A cancerous growth that arises from the two layers of the skin, the dermis and epidermis.

Sodium
A metallic element that, combined with chlorine, forms table salt. Salt is routinely added to processed foods. Excess dietary sodium is linked to causing high blood pressure, ulcers, stomach cancer, and heart disease.

Squamous cell carcinoma
A cancerous growth of the skin.

Stroke
Usually refers to a sudden vascular event that blocks critical blood flow to the brain. Cerebral strokes share similar features to a heart attack.

Sulfur amino acids
Amino acids that contain sulfur in the molecular structure, for instance, cysteine and methionine.

Synthetic retinoid
Chemically changed derivatives of vitamin A, as in trans-retinoic acid.

Systemic lupus erythematosus (SLE)
An autoimmune disease in which the immune system produces antibodies that attack the body's own DNA, protein, and structures.

Testicle
The oval male sex glands that are contained within the scrotum and store and secrete sperm.

Thea flavins
An antioxidant component found in black tea.

Thiamin
A factor of the vitamin B complex. Thiamin is found in the outer coating of many cereal grains, beans, peas, and egg yolk.

Trans-fatty acids
Formed in oils and fat from the food process called hydrogenation. Any food whose ingredient list includes partially hydrogenated vegetable oils will contain trans-fatty acids. Increased heart disease is associated with the consumption of trans-fatty acids.

Tumor
A mass of new tissue growth that is independent of its surrounding structures. Tumors have no benefits to their host and are classified as noninvasive (benign) or invasive (malignant).

Ultrasonography
An imaging technique that can measure or locate deep structures by measuring the reflection of ultrasonic waves.

Uncontrolled growth
The growth of cells that make up tissue is a tightly regulated process with many external cues. When a cell does not respond to the normal coordination of these external signals and divides on its own, this is called uncontrolled growth.

Urethra

A canal that leads from the bladder and discharges urine externally.

Urokinase

An enzyme involved in cancer progression. Compounds that impede this enzyme will do the same with cancer. Substances in green tea are known to block the enzyme urokinase.

Index

About the Author

Dr. J. Robert Hatherill is on the faculty of the University of California at Santa Barbara. He received his post-doctoral fellowship in molecular toxicology at Stanford University and doctoral degree in environmental toxicology from the University of Michigan. He is board certified in clinical chemistry by the American Society of Clinical Pathologists. He has been involved with research in environmental toxicology for 20 years and has published over 80 articles, abstracts and chapters in the field of toxicology. He is a member of the Sigma Xi and Gamma Alpha honorary societies.